Collaborative Model for
and Success for Students

Lisa A. Ruble · Nancy J. Dalrymple
John H. McGrew

Collaborative Model for Promoting Competence and Success for Students with ASD

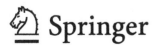

Springer

Lisa A. Ruble
University of Kentucky
Lexington, KY, USA

Nancy J. Dalrymple
Consultant
Autism Services Research Group
Bloomington, IN, USA

John H. McGrew
Department of Psychology
Indiana University-Purdue University
Indianapolis
Indianapolis, IN, USA

ISBN 978-1-4614-2331-7   e-ISBN 978-1-4614-2332-4
DOI 10.1007/978-1-4614-2332-4
Springer New York Dordrecht Heidelberg London

Library of Congress Control Number: 2012930126

Springer is part of Springer Science+Business Media (www.springer.com)

To all the children with autism spectrum disorders and their parents who have contributed to this model over the years— thank you for sharing your lives with us.

To all the teachers who cared and gave extra of themselves to perfect programs for students with ASD—thank you for your time and expertise.

To the administrators who believed in research enough to allow us to be in their schools and work with their teachers, parents, and students.

To the countless colleagues who have added their knowledge and experience to help make COMPASS work successfully—thank you for laying the foundation for greater understanding and outcomes.

Preface

COMPASS—the Collaborative Model for Promoting Competence and Success of Persons with Autism Spectrum Disorder—is a consultation framework for helping individuals with autism spectrum disorder (ASD) achieve optimal outcomes. The model represents an accumulation of more than 80 years of combined experience of the authors in collaboration with parents, teachers, administrators, and other personnel in the field. Developed and refined over 20 years, COMPASS is an excellent vehicle to systematically develop, implement, and monitor programs for students with ASD and remains one of the few experimentally tested consultation approaches associated with student progress. COMPASS is based on educational research that shows that the only empirically validated professional development model resulting in sustainable changes in teacher behavior and instruction is support that occurs within the teacher's own instructional setting.

The model described in this book was adapted originally from the work of August, Anderson, and Bloomquist and published in 1992 as the Minnesota Competence Enhancement Program. From 1978 until 1992, with both state and federal funding and under the leadership of the second author (Nancy Dalrymple) at the Indiana University (Bloomington) University Affiliated Program, the model was utilized within the UAP-based residential programs for children and youth with autism and subsequently as part of a state-wide training initiative. Over these years, as extensive data gathering continued, the model was changed as the concept of balancing risk factors with protective factors to address challenges and encourage competency was added. That concept was a key to the publication of "An Alternative View of Outcome" (Ruble & Dalrymple, 1996), which advocated for new and different ways to measure outcome by focusing on the development of competence and quality of life as central outcomes and linking these to accommodations and social and family support networks. This work helped to reaffirm the evolving model's emphasis on collaboration and building supports rather than emphasizing deficits.

Extensive field testing has continued from 1992 to the present time. In 1996 the model was used as the basis of the Autism Technical Assistance Manual for Kentucky Schools, which Lisa and Nancy authored. School systems throughout Kentucky had the opportunity to be trained with the manual, and the Kentucky

Western Education Cooperative took the lead in incorporating the model in extensive training of all their school systems over several years. This training was always specific to individual students with autism. The model was used for planning purposes, to address specific behavioral problems, and to help with transitions. Then, in 1998, the model served as the consultation framework for TRIAD at Vanderbilt University in the state of Tennessee and was renamed the Collaborative Model for Promoting Competence and Success of Persons with Autism Spectrum Disorder (COMPASS).

Since 2004, federal funding from the National Institutes of Health, National Institute of Mental Health and more recently from the NIH Challenge Grants has enabled the authors, along with current co-investigators Michael Toland, Lee Ann Jung, and Jennifer Grisham Brown from the University of Kentucky, to continue to evaluate the effectiveness of COMPASS, and to study its effectiveness via web-based technology.

Lisa A. Ruble   Lexington, KY, USA
Nancy J. Dalrymple   Bloomington, IN, USA
John H. McGrew   Indianapolis, IN, USA

Introduction

COMPASS is the first consultation model that has been verified by randomized controlled experiments and by independent evaluators to improve IEPs and associated outcomes of young students with ASD.

Everyone agrees that informed teachers, service providers, and parents need support and access to specific research-based interventions that can be individualized for each student with autism spectrum disorder (ASD). The means to this end are trained consultants, who can provide the "glue" to enable everyone to assemble and work as a team. However, these people are in short supply. This manual was developed to train consultants in assisting parents, teachers, and other service providers in working together to create positive, meaningful, effective, and personalized programs for children with autism. The model described in this manual provides a means by which a personalized approach to research-supported interventions can be used to improve the lives of students with ASD. It requires consultants who are competent about ASD and able to provide effective consultation to successfully teach individuals with autism. The goal of this manual is to prepare individuals to become such consultants.

What Is COMPASS?

Integrates Assessment and Intervention Planning

COMPASS—a collaborative model for promoting competence and success for persons with ASD—is an integrated assessment and intervention package that helps teachers develop measurable learning objectives and evidence-based teaching plans. We refer to teachers in the broadest sense and include any service provider responsible for teaching skills. Consistent with response to intervention, COMPASS is based on systematic use of progress monitoring and data-based decision making. It is a tier-three intervention support that is targeted at the individual student. Curriculum-based measurement as articulated in the IEP is used to monitor progress using goal attainment scaling. Ongoing data-based decision-making occurs by way of coaching sessions after the initial COMPASS consultation.

What Makes COMPASS Unique

COMPASS is unique from other consultation frameworks. It is the *first* consultation model that has been validated by randomized controlled experiments and by objective, trained evaluators to improve students' performance as specified in Individualized Education Programs (IEP) of young students with ASD. We believe the model is generalizable to other community based service providers such as those provided through community mental health service agencies and group home agencies.

COMPASS is consistent with educational research findings that consultation and coaching remains the only professional development method that is associated with influencing student behavior, achievement, and success.

COMPASS is also different from other models in its focus on competency development and understanding of persons in context. It underscores the fact that competencies and behaviors need to be placed in the current living experience of the individual, across school, home and community settings. It aims for measurable goals with personalized outcomes and it reflects an understanding that competencies look different across the lifespan. It is a highly individualized approach, with an emphasis on teacher and parent input and support. Lastly, it uses a consultation approach that links parents and teachers with a trained consultant/coach.

Competency Development

Competency development is based on the balance between strengths and weaknesses and when included and supported in interventions results in key quality of life outcomes. It is based on partnerships (Billington, 2006) and emphasizes identifying and building family, community, and environmental supports to promote positive outcomes. Too often standard program plans are designed to address weaknesses (isolated deficits that result from autism), rather than the whole person. Assessing the needs of the individual—along with stressors, challenges and resources, including strengths and interests—is essential when taking into account the entire person. It is vital to focus on increasing protective factors while understanding vulnerabilities and ecological stressors.

Measurable Goals and Outcomes

By focusing on measurable goals and outcomes, answers will be provided to such questions as: What will be different if we are successful? How will we know it and measure it? Details about how to teach the goal and objective are generated from a shared understanding of the balance between risk and protective factors. The factors that create the balance are the ingredients necessary for achieving competence and are unique for each individual. As a framework, this model also helps train staff to understand and support the person more effectively.

Evolving Understanding of Competence

Another focus of the model is the creation of a shared understanding that competence looks different across the lifespan of the individual. Challenges are constantly requiring new sets of skills to build competence—for the person with autism as well as their families and caregivers. People with ASD must have support from people who understand them, their personal and environmental challenges, and their personal resources in order to know how and what environmental resources will enhance learning. Too often persons with ASD are viewed as the problem because those who are trying to teach and support them do not understand their uniqueness or how their competencies may change over time.

Individualized Approach

> That was actually very helpful to me, because I don't really take the time to analyze each one of my students that much. I really don't, there isn't enough time ... but to really look helped me to see what really affected Ethan, especially in the classroom.

This statement was made by a teacher during a COMPASS consultation. A lack of time and a focus on numerous classroom and student priorities often act as environmental risk factors for generating personalized teaching objectives and strategies. That is, the very system that is tasked with helping the person with autism may unintentionally become part of the problem, placing barriers in the way of learning. COMPASS sets the stage and provides the foundation for ensuring that an individualized approach to program development is taken.

We have found it is vital to develop program plans that identify teaching strategies designed to address the individualized learning needs of each student with autism. Training approaches such as teacher workshops, in-services, and other types of professional development are important for learning about research-supported practices, but they are also insufficient. The ability to take information from the context of a workshop and apply it effectively to an individual student is often limited. Because there is not a single treatment approach that works for all students with autism, individualized assessment and decision-making is still necessary for appropriate program planning. A clear strength of consulting is its ability to help to individualize the educational program.

Training and Supporting Teachers

As more students with ASD are identified and included in schools and communities, the need for professionals and support personnel who are strongly grounded in knowledge and experience of ASD is essential. Over the years, we have learned that the most important impact we can have in consulting with parents and teachers is empowerment. We need to teach what we know, to give it away, "to teach a person to fish." A team that is empowered is one that has accurate information to make decisions and evaluate measurable outcomes after we leave. Here are some direct quotes from teachers:

- I learned more about setting up and directly teaching goals, monitoring progress and reflecting on teaching strategies and factors for success or lack thereof through watching videos taken during skill practices. Direct meta-cognition was taking place! It has carried over to my work with other students.
- I feel like it kept me on track charting his progress and moving him forward.
- I feel so much more successful as a teacher. Seeing his progress makes me proud to be a teacher.
- I feel that I have learned many strategies to try with my students. I have come to feel comfortable with some trial and error when it comes to dealing with the wide ranges of abilities and characteristics associated with teaching children with autism. I have also become more comfortable with keeping data, analyzing it, and using it to adjust instruction.
- I have been more deliberate in my teaching of specific goals. I have been encouraged to 'think out of the box' when looking for strategies.
- It made me more aware of the importance of parental involvement. This gave me confidence. There were great ideas on generating new strategies.

Consultation and Coaching: Two Different Roles, One Person

Consultation as an intervention has the potential to facilitate the training and support needed by teachers and staff. The use of consultants who can guide others in designing and monitoring the programs has the potential to improve the long-term functional outcomes of individuals with autism.

Consultation and coaching are terms often used interchangeably. But we emphasize coaching as the subsequent and necessary follow up that helps put into practice the teaching plans developed during the initial COMPASS consultation. It occurs with a focus on the context of the classroom and involves all aspects of knowledge and skill transfer that is bidirectional in its focus on plan implementation. The coach and teacher are partners who are engaged in a shared activity with a common goal. Consultation serves to set the goals and plan the strategies, and coaching helps put the plans into practice.

Supporting Parents, Caregivers, and Families

The primary environmental supports for each individual with autism are caregivers and families. They are the lifelong advocate of the person. Teachers come and go in the lives of individuals with autism. Caregivers are the ones who are truly positioned to assist others in understanding the person and advocating for services and supports. COMPASS helps provide families the opportunity to be centrally involved in planning the educational program for their loved one and a framework from which information can be shared, updated, and transferred to all professionals involved in the life of the individual. Here are some direct quotes from families:

- I feel I am able to better understand my child's educational goals at school and have gotten some useful information that I can use at home.
- His teachers have communicated more with me about how he is doing at school.
- I have learned several new methods for handling situations that may arise and new teaching methods to use at home.
- It has helped me to be able to focus on one task at a time instead of more at once.
- It has shown me how to teach my son.
- I have learned how to help my son with turn taking and answering "want" questions.

Who Should Use this Manual

This manual is designed to be used by autism specialists, early intervention and school consultants, community-based consultants, and school personnel who work with teachers or other service providers of preschool and elementary age students with autism. Although the framework applies to persons with autism across the age span, the specific protocol and forms in this manual are specialized to young children (ongoing research focuses on older children). It is assumed that an effective consultant must possess both the content knowledge of autism and also the process knowledge to apply interventions specialized for individuals with autism. It also requires training and experience in consultation. To use the manual effectively, it is assumed that certain consultation competencies and skills are in place. We strongly recommend that the reader complete the self evaluation tool provided in Chap. 3. This evaluation will assist consultants in identifying areas of need and priorities for additional learning. Also provided in Chap. 3 is a list of resources available in print and online for additional information.

Other professionals, including clinicians or behavior specialists in clinics or in other non-school based settings and other community service providers when planning services as well as families will find the manual useful as well. The COMPASS forms are helpful in sharing information about the person with others—during the start of a new program, transition to a new teacher, or introduction to a new teacher.

How to Use this Manual

The primary aim of this manual is to describe a research-supported consultation framework for young students with ASD. Research supported means the methods and tools provided in this manual have been evaluated experimentally in two randomized controlled trials. COMPASS is the first model to document that consultation can be an effective means of impacting both the quality of the IEP (e.g., goals that are measurable and specific to ASD) and the associated educational outcomes, as measured by an objective, trained observer for young students with ASD. The challenge now is how to transfer what the consultants did during COMPASS and the coaching sessions to other consultants. That is the basis of this book.

This manual is designed to be used by specialists who provide school based consultation regarding programs for young children with ASD. We recommend that the consultant read and understand the entire manual before incorporating these techniques into their own consultant work. It is crucial that the consultant adequately understands each step in the COMPASS model before moving on. This may mean the consultant will need to stop and acquire key competencies before proceeding to the next step or chapter.

Overview of this Manual

The first two chapters provide information on the importance of a consultation approach and the background and rationale for COMPASS. Chapter 3 helps the reader conduct a self-evaluation of autism knowledge and consultation process skills and includes other resources to assess for gaps in knowledge and skill. Chapter 4 discusses issues that consultants should consider (e.g., issues to consider for internal vs. external consultants) and that impact consultation outcomes. Chapter 5 provides details on evaluating the quality of IEPs as well as critical ingredients of the IEP to help ensure successful outcomes. Chapters 6–8 provide the details and protocols used during COMPASS consultation. These chapters also include sample scripts and necessary forms that are referred to within the text at the end of each chapter. The last chapter provides detailed case studies of actual COMPASS consultations. A brief description of each chapter is below.

Chapter 1 describes COMPASS as the first consultation model for persons with autism with research evidence. It describes why COMPASS is specialized for ASDs, is proactive, and is based on collaboration.

Chapter 2 explains the theoretical framework of COMPASS. Also provided is an overview of the World Health Organization's definitions of impairment, disability, and handicap and how this conceptual framework also influences COMPASS—that is, the identification of risks and protective factors—and distinguishes it from other consultation models.

Chapter 3 discusses the necessary skills for an effective COMPASS consultant. To effectively teach people with autism, it is not enough to have a consultant who is an expert in consultation: he or she must also have specific knowledge about ASD and developmental disabilities. These two aspects of consultation are presented as content knowledge and process skills. Different types of training and the competency achieved from the training are discussed. A self-evaluation form is provided for further self-study of content information.

Chapter 4 provides an overview of issues that impact effective consultation. Attention to many factors outside the immediate consultant–teacher interaction is necessary. This chapter reviews influences of the consultation process and outcomes to consider. Consultant factors and teacher factors are described as well as parent and child factors.

Chapter 5 provides more details that assist with the activities that will be described in Chaps. 7 and 8 and specifically focuses on how to write an effective individualized educational program (but the skills learned will also generalize to other types of intervention plans created and delivered by nonschool based therapists). The consultant facilitates the consultation by guiding the participants in using all the available information about the student to select objectives in communication, social, and work skills. Objectives must be well written using suggestions provided in this chapter.

Chapter 6 concentrates on Step A, the first of the two steps of the COMPASS Action Plan. It covers the activities to complete prior to conducting the consultation. Activities include gathering input from parents and teachers, or other providers using the COMPASS Challenges and Supports Forms. It also entails obtaining information from direct interactions with the child through formal and informal assessment. These activities help summarize assessment information that is used during the consultation and informs the framework for the student's personalized COMPASS profile.

Chapter 7 covers Step B of the COMPASS Action Plan. It details the mechanics of the consultation process. The IEP objectives and the teaching strategies that support competence come from the collaborative discussion of the student's strengths and challenges, both personal and environmental, that are summarized and discussed in the consultation.

Chapter 8 covers the essential components of teacher coaching. The importance of follow-up sessions from the initial COMPASS consultation is described and coaching is defined. Also provided are practical forms and a coaching protocol. The primary outcome measure of COMPASS consultation is described and instructions are provided in developing the Goal Attainment Scale (GAS) form.

Chapter 9 presents three case studies of children with ASD who were selected based on their range of presenting needs, issues, and family involvement. The first is a 4-year-old preschool child in an inclusive program who exhibited significant behavioral issues. The second is an 8-year-old third-grade child who primarily attended a general education classroom and received resource room support. The third is a first-grade student who primarily attended a special education classroom with general education support.

Teachers and Parents Comments on the Benefits of the COMPASS Consultation and Coaching Intervention

From Teachers

Benefits for Students

There has been a major improvement in social skills with both adults and peers. He is so focused on the academics and is beginning to answer questions in group settings ... and frequently he has the correct answer!

I think she has shown to many people that she is capable of things no one thought she was able to do.

He has made great progress, and I think his family benefited as well.

I think his total awareness and alertness has increased and improved due to the activities and strategies implemented. He has been drawn into the world of our classroom and has benefited from relationships with peers who have grown to understand him more as well. He has learned to respond to lots of expectations.

These new skills will help her in kindergarten and daily living.

He socializes with classmates now. Classmates have also enjoyed participating and ask to participate.

Benefits for Teachers

I have learned a lot about autism, about intervention and teaching strategies, about technology.

I found the feedback from the coaching sessions beneficial. It was encouraging to see the progress by watching the videos. Also, watching myself teach on the videos allowed me the opportunity to self-evaluate.

I realized the importance of having social skills and communication goals when working with students with autism. I felt the progress she made had to do with her working with peers in a very structured setting.

Coaching and modeling were extremely helpful—particularly techniques that are helpful when working with students who have autism.

I have learned new strategies in helping my student achieve goals, such as using peer tutoring on a higher level.

This has given me another set of eyes in my classroom. It has provided me with different strategies I can use with her when I am targeting a behavior.

From Parents

I am very pleased with the progress my son has made. By him just waving has helped me to know that he has capabilities.

Just watching the progress he has made in this short time has made life easier.

The individual work on skills has been great for my son. He continues to make small strides and for that we are blessed.

I have noticed that he will play with kids more at work when he goes with me.

She seems to be able to communicate better with less frustration.

He has grown so much in his learning, I am impressed.

I think he has made great progress in the goals that were set for him.

He has gotten a better understanding on how to act in group settings and react in an appropriate manner.

Acknowledgments

Colleagues at Indiana University:
Jack Cummings
Susan Klein
Barb Porco
IRCA staff in the early 1990s

Colleagues at the University of Louisville and the University of Kentucky:
Jim Batts
Andrea Blair
Rachel Hammond
Grace Mathai
Lonnie Sears

Other Colleagues and Autism Advocates:
Members of the Legislative Commission on Autism
MyraBeth Bundy
Susan Hepburn
Wendy Stone
Melanie Tyner Wilson

Teachers and School Administrators in Indiana, Kentucky, and Tennessee:
Judy Adams
Kathy Berg
Nancy Connor
Cheryl Cooper
Cheryl Dunn
Michele Grossman
Nancy Lovett
Debbie Plummer
Diann Shuffett

Funding Agency:

We thank our sponsor, National Institutes of Health, National Institute of Mental Health grant numbers R34MH073071 and 1RC1MH089760 for funding support. The content is solely the responsibility of the authors and does not necessarily represent the official views of the National Institute of Mental Health or the National Institutes of Health.

Contents

Chapter 1
Rationale for COMPASS

Overview: This chapter describes COMPASS as the first research-supported consultation model for young students with autism spectrum disorders (ASD). It describes why COMPASS is specialized for ASD, is proactive, and is based on collaboration.

Preschool teacher:	"It's almost like he doesn't know there is anybody or anything else going on. It's like he is in his own zone and nothing penetrates that. I'll be real honest with you: we've kind of been in survival mode. His frustration has been so high that it is just a matter of managing the tantrums. I'm at a loss. What can I do? What else can I try to replace these behaviors? What am I doing wrong?"
Parent:	"Oh my gosh! I didn't know it was that bad!"_____
Kindergarten teacher:	"I want him to be able to sit in a group and not have outbursts."
Parent:	"For so long we encouraged active participation, verbal participation, and now we are saying, 'Don't verbally respond; keep it to yourself until we say you can.'"
Kindergarten teacher:	"But as he gets older, I don't know if kids with autism understand 'Well, this is what I did when I was four, but now it's inappropriate.'"

These statements are from parents and teachers during a COMPASS consultation. They portray the frustration, differences in priorities, and, ultimately, the need for communication between parents and teachers. This manual is designed to train consultants to help caregivers, teachers, and other therapists work together to improve outcomes for young students with ASD. We wrote this manual to help consultants begin to effectively address the issues presented by these examples with the assumption that understanding the importance of building competence in persons with ASD is essential and begins with good communication as well as a common understanding of how to influence positive outcomes.

L.A. Ruble et al., *Collaborative Model for Promoting Competence and Success for Students with ASD*, DOI 10.1007/978-1-4614-2332-4_1, © Springer Science+Business Media, LLC 2012

In this chapter, we discuss the core principles that compose COMPASS:

1. COMPASS teaches consultants to measure success by considering core competencies in students with ASD, not the degree of attainment of "normal" social development.
2. COMPASS is built on a research-supported consultation framework for ASD, meaning it has been evaluated experimentally in two randomized controlled trials for young children (Ruble, Dalrymle, & McGrew, 2010a; Ruble, McGrew, Toland, Dalrymple, & Jung, 2012).
3. While COMPASS was designed to intervene with problem behaviors in students with ASD, we believe that it is most effective when used proactively to prevent problem behaviors from developing.
4. Students with ASD express certain behavioral, communication, and social needs, and COMPASS is designed especially to address the core impairments of individuals with autism.
5. COMPASS is intended to be used collaboratively, with the consultant and the consultee (the teacher or parent and child if possible) all using the model.
6. COMPASS considers the student's current services and supports and aims to improve the efficacy of those services through a dynamic and reiterative process rather than serve as a replacement process.

Measuring Success Through Competence

Every day we are faced with challenges. Our success in meeting daily challenges promotes a feeling of competence and a sense of personal well-being—along with an acceptable quality of life. Quality of life—as a goal or outcome for people with autism—is often ignored. In the past, outcomes were measured by the degree of attainment of "normal" social development and independence. Our first outcome study of young adults with autism (Ruble & Dalrymple, 1996) challenged the traditional methods researchers used to measure outcomes of adults with autism. Given this emphasis on achievement of "normal" functioning, in many ways, these studies appeared to be measuring the stability of autism over time, rather than actual clinical change associated with an intervention or outcomes. That is, social impairment, as a core defining feature of autism, remains constant over time. For example, if a person has autism in adulthood, meaning they still have social impairments, they would be judged as having a poor outcome. Instead, we offered other ways to think about and redefine outcomes. The development of competence and success was suggested as another way to consider outcome (Ruble & Dalrymple, 1996). The question is how to achieve competence. This can be challenging for us all and especially for individuals with autism spectrum disorder because they often lack the necessary skills to meet daily challenges.

Competence is defined as the ability to complete actions and tasks successfully. But we extend the definition of competency to include how well the environment helps the person be successful. The competence of a person with ASD can be enhanced by understanding how vulnerabilities interact with the environment in the face of challenges. In the COMPASS approach, competency development and enhancement requires consultants who work on behalf of individuals with ASD to empower families, service providers, teachers, and therapists through collaborative program planning and implementation.

That students need to be identified early and receive specialized services is no longer questioned by community service programs. What is less clear and more challenging is how to meet the growing and often complex needs of individuals with ASD, not only as preschoolers, but also as teenagers and adults. To assist each individual in achieving an optimal outcome and a good quality of life, more attention is needed for services research, such as how to improve the quality of services, outcomes of services, and support for teachers, clinicians, staff members, and mental health professionals in delivery of services.

Evaluating the Effectiveness of COMPASS Through Research

The need for research-supported consultation in autism is clear. The last 10 years has witnessed a shift of perception of autism spectrum disorders. Once described as a low incidence disability affecting 2 out of 10,000 children, today ASD is recognized as a relatively common developmental disability affecting 1 out of about 110 children.

Research studies during this time have also resulted in the identification of best practices for diagnostic assessment, intervention and treatment, and working with families. Because more students are being identified as having ASD, we face additional challenges—namely, the need for more autism specialists. The positive effects of intervention research have compelled the federal government, state departments, and public service agencies responsible for funding intervention to take notice because there is a recognized shortage of specialized community- or school-based personnel trained in autism (National Research Council (NRC), 2001). Moreover, because education and behavioral interventions are the primary treatments for students with autism and are most effective when received early (NRC, 2001), a lack of trained personnel has direct consequences for students with autism and their families both immediately and long-term.

The Study: From 2004 to 2007, with funding from the National Institute of Mental Health (grant number R34MH073071), we studied 35 teachers and 35 students with autism (if there was more than one student with autism in the teacher's classroom, the student was randomly picked from the group of children). Each teacher–student pair was then randomly assigned (like a flip of a coin) to the experimental group or the control group. Teachers who were chosen for the experimental group received the COMPASS consultation at the start of the school year. That consultation included the child's parent (3-h meeting) and four teacher-coaching sessions (about one-and-a-half hours per meeting every 4–6 weeks) throughout the school year. The control received no intervention from the research team. An evaluator who was unaware of the teacher–student pair group assignment evaluated the students before (at the start of the school year) and after the intervention (at the end of the school year).

The results revealed that the students whose teachers received the consultation and coaching sessions made significantly more improvements in the targeted IEP objectives. Although the control group made progress throughout the year, the COMPASS group students made progress at almost twice the rate of the comparison group children. With more recent funding from the American Recovery and Reinvestment Act (grant number RC1MH089760), we conducted a second replication study, that utilized the two groups described above (experimental and control), and a third group that was added to receive COMPASS through Web-based teacher coaching sessions, rather than face-to-face sessions. We found that the students in both of the COMPASS consultation groups (Web-based and face-to-face) made significant gains on their targeted IEP objectives compared to the control group.

To understand why COMPASS worked, we analyzed the features of the IEPs expected to change as a result of COMPASS and found that the quality of the COMPASS IEPs was higher compared to the control group (Ruble, McGrew, & Dalrymple, 2010a). That is, one of the important elements underlying effectiveness is that COMPASS helped to create higher quality IEPs, e.g., goals were more measurable and goals focused more directly on critical skills for children with autism. Chapter 5 covers information on IEPs.

Another important aspect we studied was how well COMPASS was received by both teachers and parents. Feedback from the consumers—parents, caregivers, and teachers—showed that satisfaction with the COMPASS consultation was strong. Social validity, treatment acceptability, and consumer satisfaction provide crucial information on the perceived acceptability of an intervention, a variable that plays a key role in whether an intervention is adopted. Thus, it is critical that consumers like COMPASS. A number of research-supported interventions have been rejected by consultees due to dissatisfaction with procedures (Eckert & Hintze, 2000). Social validity is discussed in more detail in Chap. 3.

Another variable that related to student progress was teachers' adherence to the recommendations from the consultation and coaching sessions, especially for the last coaching session. Teacher adherence, also called fidelity, refers to how well the teacher implemented the teaching plans. Consultants judged adherence to implementation by making an overall assessment of how many of the components from the teaching plan were implemented during instruction and by evaluating the overall quality of the implementation of the various instructional components. That is, COMPASS works better when teachers follow the consultant's suggestions. However, more research is needed to understand how coaching methods affect teacher acceptance and satisfaction as well as likelihood of following recommendations and adhering to the plans generated.

COMPASS as a Proactive Approach

Proactive collaborative program planning and effective program implementation are essential for children, youth, and adults to achieve optimal outcomes. Often, we wait until there is a problem behavior before a consultant with expertise is brought to the table. Although COMPASS was originally designed as a response to problems and used to conduct functional behavioral assessment and to develop positive behavior supports, program planning must be proactive. A proactive approach is more likely to result in expected outcomes, such as better quality and more specialized individual family service plans, individual education plans, and individual support plans.

Our research studies indicate that better program plans result in better goal attainment of the child. Further, COMPASS is helpful for transition planning, such as from early intervention to preschool; from preschool to school; from elementary to middle school. Although we have not conducted studies with older children we also expect that it will be helpful in the transition from high school to adult/vocational services. The main focus is to develop comprehensive, whole-student programs that include all people who work, live, and engage with the child.

Need for an ASD-Specific Consultation Model

There are several reasons why an autism-specific consultation model is needed. ASD is a diagnostic label that provides information about the nature of the impairments, information about the course of the disability (outcome, cause, intervention, or treatment), a basis for research, a means to receive services and information on specialized services, and, most important, a means by which parents and caregivers can organize themselves for advocacy efforts and support. This information is critical to the consultation process.

What a diagnostic label such as ASD does *not* do is identify specific teaching objectives, teaching strategies, or classroom placements. That kind of information comes from additional functional and curriculum-based assessments for program planning. Also, the teaching needs of each student are different, and what is taught, as well as how skills are taught, is unique for each child. Another challenge for students with autism is that the ability to learn—which is demonstrated by how well the student can apply skills taught in one setting, with one person, using a specific set of materials and directions—is not easily demonstrated across settings, persons, and materials, resulting in a learning weakness. Generalizing skills from one set of circumstances to another requires a team approach. It is not unusual for parents, teachers, and therapists to use different approaches and to set different teaching priorities. This becomes an environmental challenge that hinders learning.

ASD is a life-long disability, and achievement of changes in behavior may require relatively long periods of time. A time-limited consultation approach with a short-term goal of solving an immediate problem or answering a specific question may not be as effective as one with a longer-term goal of preventing problems and improving consultees' skills in problem-solving. Thus, an ongoing and systematic consultation framework is likely better and more socially valid for students who have life-long, complex disabilities like ASD.

Researchers have documented empirically supported interventions for autism (NRC, 2001). Such interventions can be categorized within one of two domains: comprehensive or focused (Odom, Boyd, Hall, & Hume, 2010). Focused interventions address specific or discrete skills. Approaches such as discrete trial training, video self-modeling, activity schedules, and social stories are examples of focused interventions. Comprehensive treatment approaches aim to improve broad areas of learning that address the core symptoms of autism. Examples of comprehensive treatment models are the Early Start Denver Model (Dawson et al., 2010), the Lovaas Model (Cohen, Amerine-Dickens, & Smith, 2006), and the TEACCH (treatment and education of autistic and related communication handicapped children) Model (Panerai, Ferrante, & Zingale, 2002). These approaches have not been compared directly with one another in an experimental way, thus we cannot say which intervention is best for each child. Further, no single specific causal mechanism that accounts for treatment progress for all individuals has been found. Instead, effective program components have been identified. Several documents are now available describing these common successful elements (National Research Council, 2001; Dawson & Osterling, 1997; Hurth, Shaw, Izeman, Whaley, & Rogers, 1999; Strain, Wolery, & Izeman, 1998) and include the following:

- Students should receive intervention at young ages.
- Intervention should be individualized to the student and family.
- Treatment should be systematic and planned and include periodic monitoring of progress and goals.
- The student should be engaged through teaching activities that foster initiative and adaptation to transitions.
- A specialized curriculum should be used that includes developmentally based programming in imitation, communication, play, and socialization.
- Treatment plans should encourage family involvement and generalization of skills to other settings.
- A functional approach to problem behaviors should be provided.

COMPASS is a framework that includes these elements. It is also a comprehensive treatment model, as it focuses on the core symptoms of autism and is tailored to the child's environment to promote the following:

- Collaboration between school personnel and parents or caregivers, in the generation of interventions.
- Linkage between assessment information and program plans.
- Prevention of problem behaviors by placing emphasis on functional skills development and environmental supports.
- The practice that teaching strategies are developed only *after* objectives is identified.

Collaborative Program Planning and Program Implementation

COMPASS aims to enhance competence of not only the student with ASD but also the person working with the student. This is done by empowering participants through a *collaborative* problem solving and program planning process that builds on comprehensive, ongoing assessments before reaching decisions. The process gathers information from both formal and informal means and from input from those who know the individual. This helps reach a consensus for building successful individualized programs.

Collaborative program planning and problem solving refers to an interactive process between people of diverse expertise and roles for the purpose of generating creative and novel solutions to mutually defined problems or questions. This approach tends to produce enhanced outcomes and solutions that are different from those produced independently (Idol, Nevin, & Paolucci-Whitcomb, 1995).

Consultation implies that the consultee (typically the teacher or parent) takes responsibility for the implementation of the intervention. But collaborators—the consultant and the consultee—share responsibility in the implementation of the program and work together from the beginning to the end—starting with assessing problems, setting goals, and designing interventions. Consultants also assume responsibility for teaching the intervention to the consultees and may share some responsibility for evaluating the outcome (Brown, Pryzwansky, & Schulte, 2006).

Including parents and caregivers as collaborators is essential. Not only is a collaborative approach preferred by teachers and parents (Freer & Watson, 1999; Sheridan & Steck, 1995), but it is also the most effective (Sheridan, Welch, & Orme, 1996). Collaborative program planning and implementation help students generalize skills from one environment to another and also helps with skill maintenance (Sheridan & Steck, 1995; Stokes & Baer, 1977; Wahler & Fox, 1981).

In addition, collaboration reinforces the intention of Part B and Part C of the federal Individuals with Disabilities Education Act (IDEA) by providing opportunities for parents and school personnel to work together. Here are direct quotes from teachers about the benefits of COMPASS for promoting collaboration:

- His general education teachers have been more excited about his progress and, therefore, have been more involved in implementing strategies which has helped his overall progress.
- It has helped get his mom involved in his education. It has helped all who work with him to focus on clear goals.
- My student has met these goals and can participate in the classroom and peers interactions successfully. It has built a more positive relationship with teachers and parent interaction.
- It has required all staff/therapists to be consistent.
- She made great progress on her goals. The videotaping and conferencing with coaches has made me more focused on her goals and how best to work with her. Plus, I worked and collaborated with a great team (OT, SLP) in developing activities related to her goals.

COMPASS as a Wrap-Around Model

COMPASS considers the child's current services and supports and aims to improve the efficacy of those services through a dynamic and iterative process rather than replacing them. In the early 1990s, the COMPASS framework was used as a process for creating a single and coordinated plan of intervention. It bridged services and supports that came from different agencies and providers, such as those from home- and community-based waiver programs for adults and students and from public schools and other adult programs, including supported employment. The need for a wrap-around model is just as necessary today as it was 20 years ago. Today, outside of their school program, students with autism receive between four and six additional types of different treatments and services provided by different professionals (Ruble & McGrew, 2007; Thomas et al., 2006). Although it is good that parents are accessing a variety of services, the unplanned interplay of interventions from multiple providers can also create problems. First, the research support from many of the interventions used is limited. And second, some providers have different treatment goals that are not coordinated with the treatment plans produced by other service providers. These differing teaching strategies and objectives may dampen outcomes. Thus, the need for single, integrated, and coordinated plans of intervention is greater than ever.

Chapter 2
Theoretical Background of COMPASS

Overview: This chapter explains the theoretical framework of COMPASS. Also provided is an overview of the World Health Organization's (WHO) definitions of impairment, disability, and handicap and how this conceptual framework influences COMPASS.

In this chapter, we describe the following:

1. The influences of behavioral, social learning theory, and mental health consultation on COMPASS.
2. How person–environment interactions which are conceptualized in COMPASS are influenced by the WHO framework of impairment, disability, and handicap.
3. Personal challenges and supports and their relationship with competence.

The overall goal of COMPASS is to provide support to the people who help and teach individuals with autism spectrum disorders (ASD) to achieve competence. Although the focus of this manual is on young students in schools, the conceptual model is well suited for older students, adolescents, and adults. The forms provided with the chapters, however, are designed for younger students. Although some of the forms may be appropriate for older individuals, the social skills assessment measures are not.

The model is based on a transactional framework (Sameroff & Fiese, 1990), and highlights the importance of the reciprocal and dynamic interactions between students and their environments. It also incorporates a multicomponent competency enhancement approach adapted from August, Anderson, & Bloomquist (1992) prevention model. Competence is assumed to operate as a protective factor that buffers the student against circumstances that contribute to failure. Because this framework assumes the development of competence results from the transaction between the person and the environment, the degree to which pathology or wellness is viewed as existing solely within the individual is reduced and the contribution of the environment is enhanced. The framework ascertains current personal and environmental challenges (risk factors) and supports (protective factors). Risk factors inhibit the

L.A. Ruble et al., *Collaborative Model for Promoting Competence and Success for Students with ASD*, DOI 10.1007/978-1-4614-2332-4_2,
© Springer Science+Business Media, LLC 2012

Fig. 2.1 Balancing
challenges and supports

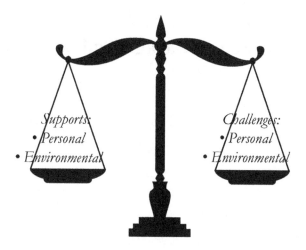

development of competence; protective factors encourage competence (August et al., 1992). Competence results when challenges are minimized by maintaining a balance in favor of supports (see Fig. 2.1).

COMPASS as a Social, Cognitive, Behavioral Model

COMPASS is influenced by multiple theories that include components of behavioral consultation, social learning theory, and the mental health model of consultation. The Behavioral Consultation Model (Bergan & Tombari, 1976) takes into account the functional relationships between behaviors and environmental contingencies and emphasizes analysis of antecedents (what occurs before a behavior) and consequences (what occurs after a behavior).

The mediating effect of internal events (thoughts and feelings) is represented by social learning theory. The COMPASS model considers aspects of social learning theory principles (Bandura, Jeffery, & Gshedos, 1975; Bandura, 1977) by acknowledging that change can be effected by a person's environment, behavior, or cognition. Most new behavior is acquired by observational learning through modeling. Models can be consultants, peers, videos, or books that depict skills. Social learning theory also takes into account consultees' own cognitions about their own self-efficacy (confidence they can perform a task) and appraisal (importance they place on completing a task or attaining a goal). Social learning theory is represented by one of the goals of COMPASS: to enhance consultees' sense of self-efficacy in solving current and future problems.

The Mental Health Model (G. Caplan, R. B. Caplan, & Erchul, 1994) builds from psychodynamic theories and stresses the importance of interpersonal relationships between consultant and consultee. Consultants need to be aware of the necessity of understanding the norms, beliefs, habits, and routines of consultees, and that ultimately, the consultee is largely responsible for putting the intervention into effect. Therefore, a collaborative approach to consultation is necessary. Consultants who assume an expert role are less likely to achieve positive outcomes compared to consultants who use key concepts of the Mental Health Model. These key factors include the following:

- The relationship between the consultant and the consultee is equitable and nonhierarchical.
- The consultant does not get involved in the personal problems of the consultee.
- The longer-term goal of consultation is to improve the functioning of the consultee for future individuals with autism whom the consultee will teach.

Distinction Between Impairment, Disability, and Handicap

Although ASD are usually considered to be lifelong (a few individuals may not carry the diagnosis over time due to clinically significant improvements), students and adults have the potential to obtain optimal outcomes that lead to productive, fulfilling, and successful lives. One may wonder how a person may achieve a successful outcome if he or she has a diagnosis of ASD. In 1980, the WHO adopted an international classification of impairment, disability, and handicap that occurs along a continuum.

- *Impairment* was defined as "any loss or abnormality of psychological, physiological, or anatomical structure or function." Impairment would relate to the diagnosis of ASD based on the disordered development of socialization, communication, and restricted repertoire of interests and repetitive patterns of behaviors.
- *Disability* was defined as "any restriction or lack [resulting from an impairment] of ability to perform an activity in the manner or within the range considered normal for a human being." The person with ASD is "disabled," for example, when s/he is unable to participate in a role or function as expected for the person's age, such as be a member of a social club at school or participate in a neighborhood play group.
- *Handicap*, on the other hand, was defined as "a disadvantage for a given individual, resulting from impairment or a disability, that limits or prevents the fulfillment of a role that is normal (depending on age, sex, and social and cultural factors) for that individual." Emphasized in this definition is the concept of "disadvantage." One disadvantage is when the person with ASD is not allowed to participate because of the attitudes or perceptions from others about ASD. For example, if a student is not taught or provided a way to communicate with others, then the person is handicapped. If the person is not allowed to use his or her communication system because it makes him or her "look different," then this attitude of others poses a handicap.

These distinctions between impairment, disability, and handicap take into account the influences between the person and his or her environment, a consideration that is important for setting expectations and developing interventions. It implies that enhancement of environmental supports are part of the therapeutic strategies that are designed to offset personal challenges or impairments that may result in disability or even handicap (Ruble & Dalrymple, 1996, 2002).

Interventions for individuals with ASD should take a two-pronged approach: one aimed at the individual and the other directed toward the environment. Interventions that focus on the individual include psychoeducational and developmental approaches. Interventions directed toward the environment include psychoeducational consultation with people or consultees (family members, teachers, employers) regarding environmental supports for the individual. The ultimate goal is for the individual with ASD to be able to participate as fully as possible and achieve his or her maximum potential and competence.

Competence Enhancement Across the Lifespan

Challenges are a part of everyday life. Depending on your present niche in life, activities requiring vocational, academic, social, communication, or leisure skills present unique challenges. Often, we fail to consider these daily challenges because we have developed the skills to master them. In fact, we often master them so well we develop a sense of competency in our skills leading to personal well-being and an acceptable quality of life for ourselves. Individuals who lack skills in meeting daily challenges fail to develop self-competence and confidence.

Competence looks different across the lifespan of the individual. The competent infant has a complex range of behaviors for meeting daily challenges. Crying, smiling, cooing, and eye contact help the infant meet daily challenges via the effects these behaviors have on caretakers. Toddlers develop early social and communicative behaviors as demonstrated in the use of language and interactive play patterns. The young student increases motor skills and cognitive abilities as evidenced in displays of independence as the student learns to negotiate challenges directly, rather than by influencing the behavior of others. Young students also face challenges in the demands for interactive play requiring that they control their emotions and understand complex social behavior such as sharing.

School provides a unique set of challenges in the development of competence. The student must adjust to being away from home and must adapt to the increased challenges of academic learning. The school setting requires that the student exhibit self-control and competencies in socialization, communication, and emotion. Play skills take the form of organized sports or may require the student to interact in peer-organized activities, such as during recess. Changes in routines also become more pronounced as students are expected to make many new transitions both at school and home. Challenges during early school years expand significantly as the student moves to adolescence and faces new and more complex demands for competency skills.

Transition to adulthood brings with it vocational decisions as well as demands for more independent living skills. The individual no longer is faced with the school routine but must now develop social and leisure activities on his or her own initiative. The social, communication, self-control, and emotional competencies continue to be refined and utilized throughout adult life. The complexity of adult relationships, including both the emotional and physical aspects, presents new and/or different challenges for individuals with an ASD. In older adults, challenges include transitions from job to job or apartment to apartment. Sometimes, older adults are presented with challenges of having to adapt their lifestyle to changes in skills brought on as a part of the aging process. The ability to cope with challenges at this stage is aided by the acquisition of competency skills early in life.

Individuals with ASD often lack the necessary competency skills to meet these daily challenges occurring across the lifespan. The competence of a person with ASD can be enhanced, however, by understanding how vulnerabilities interact and can be counterbalanced with one's personal and environmental supports (see Fig. 2.1).

Balance Between Risk and Protective Factors

The COMPASS model suggests that a balance between risk (challenges) and protective (supports) factors is an important goal. The greater the challenge for an individual, the greater the imbalance is weighted toward failure. A competent outcome to challenges depends on the balance being tipped in favor of supports. Challenges leading to poor competency include the individual's primary vulnerabilities (personal challenges) and ecological stressors (environmental challenges). Factors that protect the individual from poor competence include personal and environmental resources or supports that, when combined, produce skills to meet challenges.

Challenges

Primary challenges include biological predispositions that increase risks. Neurobiological research indicates that brain function is altered in people with ASD, leading to differences in the way they process information from the environment. The information-processing difficulties are apparent in the social and communication problems of persons with ASD as well as in their narrow range of interests and unusual sensory or motor behaviors. These vulnerabilities are apparent early in life, producing difficulties for the infant in responding competently to the social and communicative demands of the environment. The vulnerabilities lead to further problems as challenges increase with age. Comprehensive, multidisciplinary evaluations are important in identifying the primary challenges.

Adding to the personal challenges are environmental stressors. These are factors that impede competence development. Some possible stressors include misunderstandings about the individual's needs, placement in isolated settings, confusing environments, and punitive behavioral programs. A lack of trained professionals

Table 2.1 Examples of how to use individual interests to enhance other skills

An interest in music can be expanded by introducing similar music to the current repertoire.
Slowly add to the repertoire by adding varied beats, vocals, and instruments. Expand
experiences to include live music, singing, playing a keyboard, tapping rhythms, and dancing.
Music can then be used as a vehicle to share interests with others, to relax and calm down,
and for reinforcement after work

who can help plan for the life transitions of persons with ASD can produce additional
challenges. Inadequate supports for communication, social, leisure, and sensory
needs contribute to failure. Family stressors may lead also to further risk of poor
competency development in people with ASD.

Supports

While it is important to assess the personal and environmental challenges of persons
with ASD, competence enhancement focuses on the increase of protective factors.
Protective factors must balance risk factors to develop competency. During various
periods throughout a person's life, the need for protective factors will wax and wane;
however, individuals with ASD will always need help to build their personal supports. They also need a variety of environmental supports and resources to meet
their needs.

Personal supports are the strengths and interests that can produce competent
responses to challenges. Individual strengths and preferences must be identified and
then used to enhance other skills. These strengths and preferences also become the
motivators and building blocks for the development of functional life skills, the skills
essential for everyday living. Interests will change and expand as the person grows.
Relative strengths tend to remain stable, but must be enhanced. Sometimes, the interests of individuals with ASD are narrow. However, it is important to begin with current interests, gradually widening and expanding these interests. Music, puzzles, and
manipulative items, books and magazines, specific TV shows, the weather, specific
foods, riding in a car, rocking, spinning things, routines, sequences, patterns, numbers and letters, and moving—running, pacing, jumping—are samples of preferences
that individuals with ASD may demonstrate. See Table 2.1 for more ideas.

Similarly, a liking for water can be used within many activities that help meet
sensory needs. Bathing, showering, washing and rinsing dishes, watering or spraying plants, hosing/washing windows or tables, and swimming are some possible
water activities. Looking at water in falls, creeks, oceans, fountains, bottles, toilets,
and puddles can be exciting or soothing. Pouring, drinking, sipping, spraying, swirl-
ing, swishing, and splashing are a few actions to do with water. Experiencing water
by being in a shallow pool, deep pool, indoor pool, lake, or ocean broadens the
concept of swimming.

Strengths are assets on which to build a strong foundation for competency.
These must be discovered and enhanced. Sometimes, the same attribute can be

interpreted as a liability by some and a strength by others. Interpretation and the viewpoint of the observer can set the stage for competency or failure. For instance, stamina can be listed as a strength or be seen as a challenging behavior if it is called hyperactivity. Strengths might include visual and auditory memory, visual/spatial skills, desire to please, word and number recognition, gross motor skills, desire for order, self-care, and perseverance. These strengths and interests lead to competent behavior in particular areas. A person with ASD, for example, may be highly competent at completing a complex puzzle. Unfortunately, puzzle competency does not produce the social and communication competencies needed to meet the challenges of daily activities. By utilizing environmental supports, however, the unique competencies of a person with ASD can be used to develop functional skills for daily life.

Environmental supports are positive. They do not remove challenges from the lives of persons with ASD, but rather they provide the balance on which to build competency. Environmental supports must be community based, system wide, and individualized to meet each person's needs. Consistency and stability through a continuum of services as well as individual and family supports are essential. If we are going to be successful in supporting students and adults with ASD to be competent, we must collaborate across people, agencies, and government.

Some of these environmental supports are as follows:

- Family supports that include respite.
- Recreational opportunities.
- Social networks.
- Access to information and resources and meaningful programs and employment.
- Trained and knowledgeable personnel.
- Longitudinal/future planning that includes transition plans, interagency collaboration, and community access that build in stability and consistency, and promotion of choices and independence.
- Proactive, positive program components that include supports for inclusion; functional meaningful assessments; continuum of services; individual supports; and home/school collaboration. A proactive, rather than reactive, approach to problem behaviors that teaches rather than punishes.
- Positive, individualized programs that focus on using individual learning styles with visual supports, meaningful activities, appropriate pacing, and meeting sensory needs.
- Other components including teaching functional communication and social interaction skills across settings and people and teaching community skill development in collaboration with families and friends.
- Planning and developing vocational and job skills and social supports and networks are also part of positive programs.

Chapter 3
Evaluating Your Knowledge of ASD

Overview: This chapter discusses content knowledge and process skills needed by the COMPASS consultant. Various types of training and the competencies achieved from the training are discussed. A self-evaluation form is provided for further self-study.

In this chapter, we describe the following:

1. The importance of social validity.
2. The difference between content knowledge and process knowledge.
3. The three skill levels that COMPASS consultants must obtain.
4. The eight content knowledge and nine process skill competencies required of COMPASS consultants.

Before we describe the components of a COMPASS consultation, several factors must be considered. We have learned that the successes and outcomes of consultation are dependent upon the knowledge and skills of the consultant. To effectively support people with autism, it is not enough to have a consultant who is an expert in consultation: he or she must also have specific knowledge about autism spectrum disorder and developmental disabilities. We have also learned that effective consultation is based on socially valid approaches to assessment of concerns, problem solving, and identifying outcomes. That is, the more the processes, procedures, and outcomes of consultation are relevant and meaningful to the participants, the greater the likelihood of success.

This chapter focuses on influences the consultant can have on students with autism spectrum disorders. Chapter 4 covers other factors related to teacher, parent, and school influences. To ensure children with ASD reach their full potential, consultants must have the ability to carry out a socially valid consultation and apply both knowledge and process skills, as well as the ability to interact and establish a trusting, collaborative partnership with the teacher and the parent or caregiver. Thus, this chapter reviews content knowledge and process skills necessary for a COMPASS consultant and provides an overview of the concept of social validity—a critical ingredient of effective consultation.

L.A. Ruble et al., *Collaborative Model for Promoting Competence and Success for Students with ASD*, DOI 10.1007/978-1-4614-2332-4_3, © Springer Science+Business Media, LLC 2012

Social Validity

A key feature of COMPASS is its emphasis on social validity. Social validity refers to the relevance of the treatment goals, intervention procedures, and evaluation methods to the consultees (i.e., teachers and parents) (Gresham & Lopez, 1996). Consultees are empowered to decide for themselves what behaviors and skills are important. However, the COMPASS consultant shapes these perceptions by educating the consultees on outcomes in adulthood and pivotal skills that the child needs to learn to meet optimal outcomes. That is why it is important for consultants to have an enhanced understanding of outcome and longitudinal research in autism and quality of life issues.

When consultants collaborate with consultees—teachers and parents and the child with autism when appropriate and possible—on developing intervention recommendations based on their concerns, higher acceptability of the intervention plans and recommendations is the result. That is, there is a better probability of the interventions being used and adopted by teachers and parents compared to interventions of lower acceptability. Parents and teachers who increase their knowledge and understanding through consultation are more likely to accept intervention recommendations compared to parents and teachers who are not provided a means to be educated through consultation.

Content Knowledge Versus Process Knowledge

An effective COMPASS consultant must possess both content knowledge and process knowledge about autism spectrum disorder and students with ASD.

A necessary requirement for all consultants is comprehensive attainment of the subject matter (Gutkin, 1996; Sheridan, Salmon, Kratochwill, & Carrington Rotto, 1992). Content knowledge pertains to the educational and psychological base of information being shared (Gutkin, 1996). In this case, it is knowledge about ASD and developmental disabilities, educational rights of students with disabilities, assessment and IEP development, evidence based practices and programming for students with ASD, positive behavioral supports, comorbid medical problems and daily living skills, and working with parents and other school personnel.

When all personnel working with a student with ASD have a base of common knowledge on which to build, better outcomes for the student are realized. People acquire content knowledge about autism in a variety of ways, including mass media, knowing people with autism, workshops, conferences, and formal coursework. Because knowledge about ASD is constantly emerging and changing, it is important to establish ways to keep current with new knowledge as it emerges. In the forms section of this chapter, we have included resources to assist in maintaining current knowledge of research supported practices and approaches.

In addition to content knowledge, a COMPASS consultant must possess effective process skills that are utilized throughout a consultation. Process skills refer to the ability to carry out the problem-solving steps necessary to meet the goals of the consultation. While content knowledge refers to the consultant's understanding of ASD, process skills refer to the consultant's ability to actively shape understanding, teach concepts, and transfer skills to others so that teachers and parents are empowered to understand and implement program recommendations. Examples of essential process skills described by Bramlett and Murphy (1998) include competency in such core areas as: (a) social and communication skills (active listening, paraphrasing, summarizing, and reflecting feelings); (b) knowledge and application of systematic problem solving; and (c) self-reflection and self-evaluation. Competency in these areas is necessary to effectively build bridges between home and school environments, to help participants find common goals and steps to meet shared goals, and to empower participants to answer their own questions rather than need to rely on "experts." At the end of this chapter is a self-report rating scale focused on process skills.

Skill Levels Needed by COMPASS Consultants

To assist with understanding the various levels and applications of competency that a consultant should possess, a three-level approach to categorize training is offered for comparison. This approach is based on Dalrymple (1993).

- Level 1: Trainees master this competency level by identifying, discussing, and defining the concepts and skills.
- Level 2: Trainees master this competency level by participating, designing, applying, and evaluating the concepts and skills themselves.
- Level 3: Trainees master this competency level by applying, teaching, demonstrating, training, and evaluating the concepts and skills as applied to others.

These levels are illustrated in Fig. 3.1.

Level 1 is the most basic skill category and relates to the attainment of knowledge, concepts, and skills from university courses, professional development training, workshops, and conferences.

Understanding which teaching methods have research support and which ones do not is critical. The important feature for evaluating how well an intervention works is to consider its evidence. The National Professional Development Center on Autism Spectrum Disorders (NPDCASD) defines evidence-based practice as methods that have been reported in peer-reviewed scientific journals using (a) randomized or quasi-experimental design studies, such as two high-quality experimental or quasi-experimental group design studies; or (b) single-subject design studies, such as three different investigators or research groups who have conducted five high-quality single subject design studies, or (c) a combination of evidence, such as one high-quality randomized or quasi-experimental group design study and three

Fig. 3.1 Skill levels needed
by the COMPASS consultant

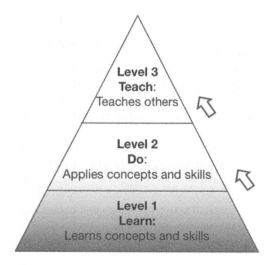

high-quality single subject design studies conducted by at least three different investigators or research groups (across the group and single subject design studies). Table 3.1 lists the evidence-based practices identified by the NPDCASD.

Establishing Level 1 competencies, including knowledge of evidence based practices, can be accomplished in several ways. For teachers of children with autism, obtaining competencies in the area of autism is a practice standard. In 2009, the National Council for Accreditation of Teacher Education (NCATE) endorsed performance-based standards in autism developed by the Council for Exceptional Children. The standards are categorized into initial and advanced knowledge/ skill sets and are online at http://www.cec.sped.org/Content/NavigationMenu/ ProfessionalDevelopment/ProfessionalStandards/default.htm—Standards. As a result of requirements for competencies in autism, a number of helpful online sources have been made available that can facilitate assessment of learning needs and resources to acquire Level 1 competencies. As more research is conducted, the list of evidence based practices will change and grow. At the time of this writing this list is current, but the Web site ukautism.org will be maintained with an up-to-date description of Web sites that provide information on research supported practices in autism.

- The first comes from the National Professional Development Center on Autism Spectrum Disorders at the Frank Porter Graham Child Development Institute. Information on research-supported teaching methods is available at http:// autismpdc.fpg.unc.edu/content/briefs. Each of these treatment methods represents a focused intervention designed to target a specific skill. An overview of the method is provided, followed by step-by-step instructions for implementation, an implementation checklist, and a description of the evidence base (see Table 3.1).

Table 3.1 Evidence-based practices for children and youth with ASD[a]

- Antecedent-based interventions (ABI)
- Computer-aided instruction
- Differential reinforcement
- Discrete trial training
- Extinction
- Functional behavior assessment
- Functional communication training
- Naturalistic intervention
- Parent-implemented interventions
- Peer-mediated instruction and intervention
- Picture exchange communication system (PECS)
- Pivotal response training
- Prompting
- Reinforcement
- Response interruption/redirection
- Self-management
- Social narratives
- Social skills groups
- Speech-generating devices/VOCA
- Structured work systems
- Task analysis
- Time delay
- Video modeling
- Visual supports

[a]From the National Professional Development Center on Autism Spectrum Disorders

Other valuable resources are accessible such as the National Professional Development Center on Autism Spectrum Disorders' course content for foundation of ASD, available at http://autismpdc.fpg.unc.edu/content/foundations-autism-spectrum-disorders-online-course-content. A reading list and PowerPoint presentation are available for eight areas that include understanding ASD, characteristics of ASD, assessment of ASD, guiding principles for working with children and youth with ASD, factors that impact learning, instructional strategies and learning environments, communication and social interventions, and increasing positive behavior.

- A second online resource comes from the Ohio Center for Autism and Low Incidence at http://www.autisminternetmodules.org. Information on recognizing autism and on strategies for the home, the classroom, the workplace, and the community is provided through videos and text. Each module has a list of objectives, a definition of the intervention, a summary, references, and a self-assessment.
- A third online resource, from the Interactive Collaborative Autism Network, can be found at http://www.autismnetwork.org/modules/index.html. This comprehensive online resource represents a collaborative effort among three states for

training in autism spectrum disorders. The site provides information on characteristics of autism, functional behavioral assessment, and academic, behavioral, communication, environmental, sensory, and social interventions. Each learning module has an introduction, lecture, quiz, frequently asked questions, and references.

Once Level 1 competencies are achieved and the learner can identify, discuss, and define the concepts and skills indicated in the key content areas, the learner then focuses on Level 2 competencies. At this second level, the learner applies the knowledge and concepts obtained from Level 1 using a variety of approaches. Level 2 competency includes participating, designing, applying, and evaluating the concepts and skills depicted by discussing, reviewing, analyzing, describing, and explaining content areas through verbal, written, and other means. Level 2 content knowledge is demonstrated through observable actions that might include activities such as discussing current theories of autism, conducting a functional behavioral assessment, writing measurable IEP objectives, analyzing and critiquing one's own teaching skills, etc. The ability to model, provide performance feedback, and direct teaching are Level 2 skills that are important for learning how to transfer knowledge and skills to another person. Our experience tells us that achievement of Level 1 skills alone is not sufficient and does not lead automatically to competency of Level 2 skills. Further, attainment of Level 2 skills does not necessarily lead to accomplishment of Level 3 skills. Supervised practice and feedback are suggested ways to develop Level 2 skills.

Level 3 competencies emphasize the ability to teach and train others in the content described in Levels 1 and 2 categories. To effectively consult with others regarding students with ASD, a person should be able to meet Levels 1, 2, and 3 competencies. Level 3 competency is based on the ability to apply, teach, demonstrate, and train concepts and skills to others. Examples of Level 3 competencies include the ability to teach others about the characteristics and causes of autism, to train others to assess the learning strengths and weaknesses of individuals with autism and develop teaching plans based on assessment information, and to teach others to teach individuals with autism using research-supported methods. The ability to transfer such knowledge and skills to other professionals requires specialized process skills described in the next section.

Competencies for a COMPASS Consultant

Content Knowledge

A lot has already been said about competencies in autism. The Level 1 competencies we suggest for a COMPASS consultant are listed in Table 3.2. Eight areas of competency are recommended and range from understanding the basics on developmental disabilities, to inclusion and public policy, to assessment and intervention

Table 3.2 The COMPASS consultant must be competent in eight key areas

- Developmental disabilities and ASD
- Inclusion, public policy, and the service system
- Assessment and IEP development for students with ASD
- Programming for students with ASD
- Positive behavior support
- Medical needs and daily living skills
- Collaboration with parents
- Involvement with school personnel

Table 3.3 The COMPASS consultant must be competent in nine key process areas

- Explaining the purpose and outlining the agenda
- Clarifying questions and concerns
- Keeping the group moving and focused
- Involving all participants
- Valuing all participants' input
- Questioning members effectively to draw ideas from group
- Collaborating with parents
- Being flexible enough to include unexpected information
- Summarizing as group moves along

planning and implementation, to medical issues, and collaborating with families and school personnel (Dalrymple, 1993). A more detailed list of items within these domains and a self-report rating questionnaire are provided at the end of this chapter. You should use this questionnaire to identify areas of further study and concentration. The items in the self-report questionnaire are not meant to be comprehensive, but are meant to represent minimal areas of knowledge required. To address gaps in knowledge identified by the self-report questionnaire, it is necessary for the reader to seek out sources of training, such as the online sources of training described earlier. Also, a reading list associated with the self-evaluation form is provided at the end of the chapter.

Process Skills

The ability to transfer skills and knowledge from the COMPASS consultant to the teacher is facilitated by nine key process skills depicted in Table 3.3. Consultation begins with a clear explanation of the purpose and expected outcomes and ends with a mutually defined plan of action. In between these two actions are the active listening and group management skills that ensure that participants are purposefully and meaningfully involved and that the agenda for the consultation is successfully met. As the information is shared about the child's strengths and weaknesses and teacher and parent concerns, the consultant asks questions and clarifies comments to ensure that all participants have a common understanding. The consultant maintains awareness of the time spent on various components of the consultation and gently transitions from one area to another by summarizing information that keeps the group moving and the topic focused. This is done by acknowledging comments and concerns and reminding the group of the task at hand. If some participants are particularly domineering and others passive, the consultant directs nonthreatening open-ended questions and elicits input from the quiet participants. Participants' viewpoints are valued and not judged by using active listening techniques that include paying attention, staying on topic and avoiding distractions, asking questions or making comments about the topic, and reflecting the person's feelings.

Paying attention is demonstrated through providing undivided attention. This can include looking at the speaker, using an open and inviting posture, "listening" to the speaker's body language and the body language of the other participants, communicating attentive body language through gestures, nods, and facial expressions, using minimal encouragers such as "yes" and "uh huh," and a tone of voice that communicates interest.

Reflecting what is said includes paraphrasing and asking clarification questions. As the consultant, it is important to maintain awareness of the impact statements have on the participants and you. In emotionally charged communications, the consultant may listen for feelings. Rather than paraphrase what was said, the consultant may describe the underlying emotion involved.

Although COMPASS is best applied as a proactive intervention planning process, it may be used during times of conflict between the parents and school personnel. Under such conditions, it is important to keep in mind that individuals in conflict may contradict each another. We have found, however, that this is less likely to occur when focus is maintained on the child and agreement is made at the outset that the purpose of the consultation is to help the child. Remind the participants that they are all there because they care about the child and are all critical to finding, agreeing on, and implementing solutions. They are not part of the problem, but part of the solution, and a consistent, unified approach is necessary. Cognitive reframing is helpful in maintaining a positive tone. If everyone is focused on understanding the child and his/her needs, an atmosphere of cooperation and collaboration can be created. This increases the possibility of true collaboration and conflict resolution.

In summary, possessing knowledge of evidence-based practices in autism is necessary for being a good consultant, but this knowledge alone is not sufficient to help a student with ASD realize optimal outcomes. In addition to possessing knowledge, an effective consultant must be able to transfer skills to others. This transfer happens through the use of effective process skills. Chapter 4 presents additional information on issues that a consultant should consider. Chapter 5 describes effective IEPs for students with autism. Together, Chaps. 3–5 provide the foundations for applying the COMPASS Consultation Action Plan and the COMPASS Coaching Protocol is presented in Chaps. 6–8.

Appendix A   Self-Evaluation of Competencies for Consultants and People Teaching Students with Autism Spectrum Disorders

By completing this checklist, you can assess your areas of strengths and determine areas where you may need to gain more knowledge and experience. A resource list of readings is provided for each of the areas. References refer to specific readings for that competency. The list of readings is not comprehensive. Consultants should seek out additional resources as needed.

Please rate each skill from 1 ("not very much/well") to 4 ("very much/well") based on where you believe your skills are at the present time.

1	2	3	4
Not very much/well			Very much/well

Area 1: Developmental Disabilities and ASD

	1	2	3	4
Knowledge about general child development	1	2	3	4
Motor skills: fine motor, gross motor, perceptual motor (National Research Council, 2001a)	1	2	3	4
Communication: receptive, expressive, social (National Research Council, 2001b)	1	2	3	4
Social skills and play (National Research Council, 2001c)	1	2	3	4
Cognitive development (National Research Council, 2001d)	1	2	3	4
Adaptive behavior (self-care, community skills, functional skills) (National Research Council, 2001e)	1	2	3	4
Affective/emotional/behavior development (National Research Council, 2001f)	1	2	3	4
Knowledge about causes, definitions, and functional implication of developmental disabilities	1	2	3	4
Can describe various causes of developmental disabilities (Lord & Spence, 2006)	1	2	3	4
Can name several developmental disabilities (Lord & Spence, 2006)	1	2	3	4
Can distinguish between terms: disease, impairment, disability, handicap, birth defect, developmental disability (Heward, 2009)	1	2	3	4
Can discuss the functional definition for developmental disability (National Institutes of Health (2011))	1	2	3	4
Knowledge about the characteristics of ASD and criteria used to diagnose ASD (Quill, 2000a, 2000b)	1	2	3	4
Characteristics of ASD and how these affect the individual (Lord & Spence, 2006)	1	2	3	4
Strategies for intervention with core deficits of ASD individually identified (Pretzel & Cox, 2008)	1	2	3	4
Knowledge of current theories about the causes of ASD (Hale & Tager-Flusberg, 2005; Bebko & Ricciuti, 2000; López, Leekam, & Arts, 2008; Grandin, 2006a)	1	2	3	4

1	2	3	4
Not very much/well			Very much/well

Knowledge of historical controversies about the causes of ASD (Eggertson, 2010; Fombonne, 2003)	1	2	3	4
Knowledge of the work of significant contributors to the field of ASD	1	2	3	4
Early pioneers (Wing, 1997; Grandin, 2006b)	1	2	3	4
People with ASD (Grandin, 2006b)	1	2	3	4
Field of communication (National Professional Development Center on Autism Spectrum Disorders, 2008a)	1	2	3	4
Field of medical interventions (IAN Community, 2011)	1	2	3	4
Field of educational intervention (National Professional Development Center on Autism Spectrum Disorders, 2008b; Autism Spectrum Disorder Foundation, 2007)	1	2	3	4
Field of psychological intervention (Grandin, 2006b; Howlin, 2003)	1	2	3	4
Knowledge of factors contributing to quality of life for individuals with ASD (Ruble & Dalrymple, 1996)	1	2	3	4

Area II: Inclusion, Public Policy, and the Service System

Knowledge of major legislation regarding education and rights of students with disabilities (Heward, 2009)	1	2	3	4
Knowledge of structure and function of state and local agencies and groups that serve or advocate for individuals with disabilities (Heward, 2009)	1	2	3	4
Knowledge of current concepts that are important in education and rights of individuals with disabilities (inclusion, supported services) (Heward, 2009; Nickels, 1996)	1	2	3	4

Area III: Assessment and IEP Development for Students with ASD

Knowledge of the value of collaboration across disciplines and situational assessments in diagnosis and educational planning (Smith, Slattery, & Knopp, 1993)	1	2	3	4
Knowledge of effective use of assessment procedures with individuals with ASD (Pretzel & Cox, 2008)	1	2	3	4
Knowledge of the use of assessment information to design individual objectives that relate to current skills, functional needs, age-appropriate curriculum, state academic content standards, and federal guidelines (Smith et al., 1993; Burns, 2001)	1	2	3	4

1	2	3	4
Not very much/well			Very much/well

Area IV: Programming for Students with ASD

Knowledge of evidence-based strategies for teaching students with ASD (The National Professional Development Center on Autism Spectrum Disorders)	1	2	3	4
Knowledge of ways to design and structure teaching environments and supports that best accommodate the needs of students with ASD (Quill, 2000b; Heward, 2009)	1	2	3	4
Knowledge of how to design individual teaching strategies, interventions, and activities to assure success for each IEP objective (Jung, Gomez, Baird, & Galyon-Keramidas, 2008; Ruble et al., 2010b)	1	2	3	4
Knowledge of how to design and maintain a useful, functional data-keeping system relevant to IEP objectives (Jung et al., 2008)	1	2	3	4
Knowledge of how to implement positive teaching strategies when implementing educational activities (positive reinforcement, fading of prompts, shaping and reinforcing successive approximations, task analysis, chaining, desensitization, incidental teaching, relaxation, rehearsal, generalization) (Heward 2009a; Nounopoulos, Ruble & Mathai, 2009; Roselione, 2007)	1	2	3	4
Knowledge of how to account for individual learning challenges such as generalization difficulties, over-selectivity, processing style, expressive and receptive communication difficulties, sensory and perceptual problems, and social interaction difficulties (Quill, 2000a, 2000b)	1	2	3	4
Knowledge of communication strategies that effectively enhance competence for individuals with ASD (Quill, 2000a, 2000b)	1	2	3	4
Knowledge of social interaction strategies that effectively enhance inclusion and self-esteem for individuals with ASD (Quill, 2000a, 2000b)	1	2	3	4
Knowledge of current teaching programs or strategies and when and how to effectively use these for individual students (e.g., applied behavior analysis, structured teaching, incidental teaching) (Quill, 2000b)	1	2	3	4

Area V: Positive Behavior Support

Knowledge of analysis of behavioral challenges encountered by students with ASD (Quill, 2000; Nounopoulos et al., 2009)	1	2	3	4
Knowledge of a functional assessment of behavior and understanding the purposes of behavior (Koegel & Koegel, 2006)	1	2	3	4
Knowledge of skills that can be taught to replace challenging behavior (Heward, 2009a)	1	2	3	4
Knowledge of data keeping and adjustments to a behavioral program (National Professional Development Center on Autism Spectrum Disorders, 2008c)	1	2	3	4

1	2	3	4
Not very much/well			Very much/well

Area VI: Medical Needs and Daily Living Skills

Knowledge of common medical issues encountered by individuals with ASD (Thompson, 2007)	1	2	3	4
Knowledge of common challenges of daily living encountered by individuals with ASD (sleeping, eating, toileting, understanding danger) (Autism Services Research Group, 2004)	1	2	3	4

Area VII: Collaboration with Parents

Knowledge of ways to involve parents as partners in the educational process (Wetherby & Prizant, 2000)	1	2	3	4
Knowledge of ways to effectively share information and problem solve throughout the school year (Nickels, 1996)	1	2	3	4

Area VIII: Involvement with School Personnel

Knowledge of ways to inform staff members about students with ASD and how they can be collaborative partners in the education of the students (Ruble & Akshoomoff, 2010; Ruble & Dalrymple, 2002; Schwartz, Shanley, Gerver, & O'Cummings)	1	2	3	4
Knowledge of ways to share information and build a collaborative team for a student with ASD across all team members who work with the student (Ruble & Dalrymple, 2002; Snell & Janney, 2000)	1	2	3	4
Knowledge of ways to build a team within the classroom and interface with teaching assistants to benefit students with ASD (Walther-Thomas, Bryant, & Land, 1996)	1	2	3	4

Appendix B   Self-Evaluation of Process Skills Necessary for Level III COMPASS Consultation

By completing this checklist, you can assess your areas of strength and determine areas where you may need to gain more knowledge and experience. Suggested resources for more information on consultation and coaching with teachers and families, including culturally diverse families, are provided at the end of this questionnaire. Chapters 3 and 7 cover each of these areas.

Please rate each skill from 1 ("not very much/well") to 4 ("very much/well") based on where you believe your skills are at the present time.

1	2	3	4
Not very much/well			Very much/well

Area 1: Explaining the Purpose and Outlining the Agenda

Provide an overview and explanation of COMPASS	1	2	3	4
Explain the purpose/outcomes of COMPASS consultation	1	2	3	4
Provide an overview of best practices in teaching children with autism	1	2	3	4

Area 2: Clarifying Questions and Concerns

Ask open-ended questions	1	2	3	4
Paraphrase what is said	1	2	3	4
"Listen" for feelings	1	2	3	4

Area 3: Keeping the Group Moving and Focused

Attend to the time involved for each aspect of the consultation and monitor allotted time throughout consultation	1	2	3	4
Allow enough time for information to be shared, but not too much time that all activities are not completed	1	2	3	4
Gently redirect conversations that stray from the goal of the activity	1	2	3	4

Area 4: Involving All Participants

Steer dominant participants to listen	1	2	3	4
Ask open-ended questions and seek information from quiet participants	1	2	3	4
Summarize concerns as a topic area closes	1	2	3	4

1	2	3	4
Not very much/well			Very much/well

Area 5: Valuing All Participants' Input

Remain nonjudgmental	1	2	3	4
Use attentive and open body posture	1	2	3	4
Use gestures, nods, and facial expressions to communicate attending	1	2	3	4
Use minimal encouragers	1	2	3	4
Use a tone of voice that communicates interest	1	2	3	4

Area 6: Demonstrating Sensitivity and Responsivity to Culturally Diverse Families and Teachers

Identify colloquialisms used by families or teachers that may impact consultation	1	2	3	4
Provide written information to parents in their language of origin	1	2	3	4
Use alternative formats to communicate with family members who experience disability	1	2	3	4
Avoid imposing one's own values that may conflict or be inconsistent with those of other cultures or ethnic groups	1	2	3	4
Demonstrate understanding that traditional approaches to disciplining children are influenced by family culture	1	2	3	4
Be able to adapt many evidence-based approaches with children and their families from culturally and linguistically diverse groups	1	2	3	4
Demonstrate that family/parents are the ultimate decision makers for services and supports for their child	1	2	3	4

Area 7: Questioning Members Effectively to Draw Ideas from Group

Ask questions that relate to the topic and are open-ended	1	2	3	4
Use Socratic questioning techniques	1	2	3	4
Avoid giving answers and instead ask questions	1	2	3	4
Avoid acting as "expert"	1	2	3	4

Area 8: Being Flexible Enough to include Unexpected Information

Adjust allotted time to address issues or concerns that arise	1	2	3	4
Prioritize time to address unexpected information	1	2	3	4
Validate concerns	1	2	3	4

1	2	3	4
Not very much/well			Very much/well

Area 9: Summarizing as Group Moves Along

Summarize information before moving on to new topic or area of discussion	1	2	3	4
Rephrase information in your own words	1	2	3	4

Area 10: Concluding with a Plan for Further Action

Develop clear action plan for follow-up	1	2	3	4
Check everyone's understanding of plan and clarify any questions or ambiguities	1	2	3	4

Chapter 4
Other Considerations for the Consultant

Overview: Effective consultation requires attention to many factors outside the immediate consultant–teacher interaction. Chapter 4 reviews influences on the consultation and coaching processes and identifies outcomes to consider. Consultant factor and teacher factors are described, as well as parent and student factors.

In this chapter, we describe the following:

1. A framework for teacher training
2. Consultant characteristics that impact consultation
3. Teacher characteristics that impact consultation
4. Parent and student considerations

For decades, educational researchers have searched for answers to the question "What makes good teachers?" Some teachers are naturals. They make teaching look easy—keeping a classroom of students engaged and on task. But most teachers have to learn ways to instruct a classroom of students, adapt and modify teaching strategies and materials, and manage student behavior effectively. The effort to stay current and learn new teaching methods based on research is more difficult than ever today because teachers are responsible for all learners—those with and without disabilities. As more and more information becomes available, sorting through information on research-supported practices can be overwhelming. Assuring that all students learn is a daunting task and requires ongoing commitment to professional development. But as we have noted in Chap. 3, professional development is not enough for optimal outcomes. The focus of this chapter is to describe the multiple factors that influence outcomes, including consultant, teacher, and student factors. We begin with a description of a theoretical model for teacher training.

L.A. Ruble et al., *Collaborative Model for Promoting Competence and Success for Students with ASD*, DOI 10.1007/978-1-4614-2332-4_4,
© Springer Science+Business Media, LLC 2012

work for Teacher Training

... uiat shows the various sources of influence on teacher training outcomes is provided in Fig. 4.1 (adapted from Sparks, 1988). It is helpful to be aware of this model because consultation is a complex task, and Fig. 4.1 shows the many pieces of the puzzle that must be considered. We have selected parts of the model that we believe affect teacher and student outcomes and used these parts in our development of COMPASS (future applied research will continue to study, adapt, and refine the model). A brief explanation of each of the pieces is provided. In this model, outcome variables—the most important part of the framework, are referred to as product variables. Product variables can include outcomes that relate to the teacher, parent, or student. For COMPASS, we selected goal attainment scaling (GAS) as the primary student outcome. GAS is a good alternative for measuring child-specific educational outcomes when goals are individualized.

- Teacher outcomes might include the teacher's instructional methods or style, the teacher's sense of self efficacy or competence, or the quality of the student's individual education program (IEP) plan. COMPASS is designed to improve IEP quality, which is thought to act as a mediating variable for student outcome. That is, IEP quality helped explain student outcomes because we found a positive correlation with student goal attainment scores. These variables in Fig. 4.1 serve as examples of areas that might change as a result of consultation, but other outcomes can also be targeted.

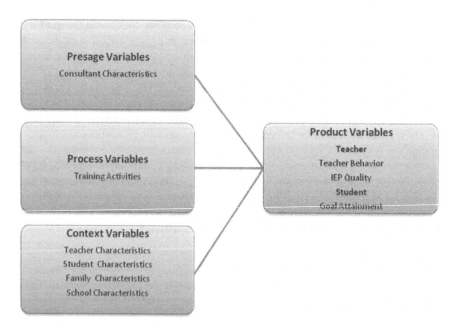

Fig. 4.1 Framework for teacher training

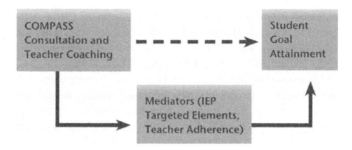

Fig. 4.2 COMPASS mediation model tested

- Parent or caregiver outcomes might include parent and teacher alliance or the amount of stress the parent feels. One parent told us that her stress was reduced because it was reassuring to know that a knowledgeable team was actively involved and working with her child. More research is needed on secondary effects of COMPASS on parents and caregivers.
- Recall that student outcomes are the primary focus of COMPASS. GAS serves as the primary mode of curriculum-based assessment of student attainment of IEP objectives and COMPASS outcome. Chapter 8 includes information on how we measured this outcome and developed the GAS Form. Figure 4.2 shows the COMPASS mediation model that we tested (Ruble, Dalrymple, & McGrew, 2010a) using parts described in Fig. 4.1. A mediator is a variable that helps explain the relationship between two other variables. In our model we examined only two possible mediators—or as we call them, active ingredients—of the COMPASS intervention: (1) the quality of the student's IEP and (2) teacher adherence to the teaching plans. IEP quality is described in more detail in Chap. 5. Teacher adherence is covered in Chap. 7.

It is important to have a theoretical model to test because it helps us to carefully and systematically examine what influences outcomes. If we study the model predictions and obtain the expected results, we can then make sure to include aspects that have been found to be important for positive student learning in our interventions. If we don't find the expected results, then we know what we should exclude and what factors are not necessarily important and influential. Of course, this assumes that we have all the relevant and important variables in the model. When comparing the model we tested in Fig. 4.2 with the original model in Fig. 4.1, it is clear that we examined a limited set of potential variables that could influence outcomes. More research on those other potential factors is needed. The following section discusses the other factors in more detail.

Three categories of influences on outcomes are proposed in the original model in Fig. 4.1. The first is *presage variables*, which refer to the characteristics of the consultant that are expected to have influence on outcome variables. Throughout this manual information on important consultant factors is provided (e.g., level 1 competence). COMPASS was developed based on current theories of effective consultation and communication between adult collaborators and learners. Chapters 6–8 provide specific steps to help ensure that a successfully collaborative partnership is established with the teacher and parent. However, other influences from a consultant have to be taken into account and are described further in this chapter.

Additional features that influence consultation effectiveness come from *process variables* as well as *context variables*. The process variables are the activities we discuss in Chaps. 6–8 specifically. These variables represent the elements of the COMPASS consultation package (e.g., respectful communication, empathic listening, appropriate goal setting). Context variables include teacher (e.g., autism knowledge), student (i.e., language ability), family (e.g., economic resources), and school characteristics (e.g., supportive special education director) that influence consultation outcomes. As an example, preliminary findings from our COMPASS consultation intervention research analyzed data on some of these factors and how well they predicted student goal attainment outcomes. Although the findings need to be replicated in a different sample, we found that the following context variables of the student and teacher predicted outcomes.

For the student, IQ level, language ability, and autism severity were predictors of his or her outcomes. But only IQ exhibited predictive power to explain student outcomes beyond the contribution of the COMPASS consultation intervention. In other words, the consultation was able to account for and adapt to differences in language and autism severity so that outcomes remained similar.

For teacher-related context variables, we found that teacher engagement predicted child outcomes beyond the effects of the COMPASS intervention. For this reason, we included the Teacher Engagement Scale in the forms section in Chap. 8. Improving the instructional engagement of teachers may be another active ingredient that needs to be studied further. One other teacher context variable identified as important was teacher exhaustion. Surprisingly, we found that students whose teachers reported more exhaustion, which is representative of burnout, made less progress. More research is clearly needed to better understand the impact of burnout in teacher instruction and student outcome.

Together, these variables are thought to have impact on the product or outcomes of consultation. The focus of the rest of the chapter is to provide general descriptions of issues that consultants should consider.

Consultant Characteristics: External Vs. Internal Consultants

Consultants can be internal or external to a school, and each has advantages and disadvantages. Internal consultants might be autism specialists who have completed additional professional development training and workshops and developed expertise in this particular area. Large school systems often have designated autism experts on staff. External consultants, on the other hand, might come from local, regional, state, or out-of-state areas. Some state Departments of Special Education have regional consultants who are designated to work in certain school districts and counties. The work reported in this manual is based on COMPASS consultants who were external to the school system. External consultants are more common for schools located in rural areas. Particular issues should be considered depending on whether the role of a consultant is external or internal to the organization. Issues to consider include entry, confidentiality, evaluation of the teacher, and willingness to participate in consultation.

Entry

Acceptance of the consultant is easier to achieve for internal rather than external consultants. An advantage of the internal consultant is that the (s)he is likely to have more information about the challenges and resources and to be better able to identify supports and the feasibility of the consultation plans that the teacher may not consider. Internal consultants may be better able to meet more frequently with the teacher and obtain data more easily and on a more continuous basis. They may also have more information about the student, the parents, and the teacher that may impact outcomes.

There are some disadvantages for internal consultants, however. One disadvantage may be a lack of role clarity. The consultant may have other responsibilities and titles that may affect the relationship with the teacher and, as a result, dampen outcomes. Teachers who are peers, for example, may be less likely to request or accept help and be more defensive and less inclined to provide data on student progress if the student is having difficulty achieving set goals. A second consideration is that internal consultants may have difficulty making demands on administrators or may have supervisory status over the teacher. They also may be in a position to more likely consult with or involve administrators or those with supervisory responsibility or other power figures. Another concern is that teachers may be reluctant to engage the internal consultant because of worries of how to terminate the consultation and what effects that might have on ongoing relationships.

Thus, it is essential that the role of the consultant be made explicit and be distinguished from other roles played within the organization. For example, a school psychologist who normally provides therapeutic services to students may want to explain that the role of consultant is different from that of therapist, and that the goal is not for the school psychologist/consultant to take over and assume responsibility of therapy for the student. A helpful summary of the relative advantages and disadvantages for internal and external consultants is provided by Brown, Pryzwansky, and Schulte (2006).

Similar to internal consultants, outside consultants also face unique advantages and disadvantages. Disadvantages include less knowledge about the history of the issues or contextual factors and resources and more difficulty identifying helpful linkages to address any problems that may arise. Another disadvantage is a dependency on information as given by the teacher, rather than from multiple sources that can help clarify or confirm the problem.

However, there also are several potential advantages for an external consultant. First, teachers may find it easier to share information with an external consultant and may be less defensive if a child is not making progress or recommendations are not being followed. An outsider may be afforded a perception as "expert" compared to a familiar internal consultant and thus, have more influence. An external consultant may also be better positioned to test how ready a teacher is to make change and obtain resources for change because of the lack of familiarity of the consultant to the system; an external consultant brings a wider perspective that may be helpful for leveraging participation and commitment of resources for making change.

Confidentiality

Establishing an effective relationship with the teacher is integral to consultation. Understanding the role of the teacher in the classroom and as part of the school is an active goal of the consultant. Also critical is the establishment of a nonhierarchical relationship within which issues and concerns can be discussed openly and in a nonjudgmental fashion. Equally and extremely important is dealing with confidentiality—explicitly, clearly, and repeatedly. It is necessary for the teacher to know that consultation will not be discussed with others, including supervisors, principals, or any superiors. For external consultants, this will be an easier objective to meet; for internal consultants, it may be more difficult, especially if the consultant is part of the administrative structure. In this latter case, the consultant needs to be aware of his/her authority over the consultee and limitations that follow. Under these circumstances, there may be barriers to discussing the questions and issues with the teacher because the consultation may not viewed by the teacher as strictly confidential or voluntary and may be used as part of teacher evaluation. Because it is not possible to establish a coordinated, nonhierarchical relationship, teachers may be more reluctant to open up and share information that will help the consultant to be more aware of the teacher's perceptions, roles, and feelings. Thus, each issue— confidentiality, evaluation, and willingness to participate should be discussed with the teacher.

Evaluation of the Teacher

Internal consultants must take great care to assure administrators that information shared during the consultation remains confidential. Potential conflicts of interest should be anticipated and discussed up front with the teacher and with administrators. Internal consultants likely take on several roles in schools. A school psychologist, for example, may conduct evaluation of students for special education services. They may also be responsible for assisting teachers with students with behavioral problems. Information learned during consultation may impact decision-making about referrals for evaluation. Supervisors may seek out consultants for feedback on teacher performance. Issues related to teacher evaluation that come from internal or external consultants should be discussed up front and communicated to all for clear understanding.

Willingness of Teacher to Participate

Early in consultation research, it was assumed that the consultee had the power to decide whether or not to initiate consultation. Today, the picture is different. Often, it is the decision of a team, parent, or supervisor to initiate and seek consultation from a person external or internal to the system. It can be argued that an internal consultant shares in the responsibility for the student, as both the teacher and the consultant are employees of the same system. For nonvoluntary consultation, teachers may need to assess their own willingness to enter into the consultation process. The consultant needs to consider the balance in time and effort required by the teacher to be part of the process, the use of social influence strategies, and the transfer of ownership of the problem during the consultation process. Teachers who are better informed of the consultation process and expected outcomes will be more aware, and thus likely more committed, to the process, expectations, and outcomes.

Teacher Characteristics

Teachers have several activities that they must participate in that either directly or indirectly relates to student instruction. A variety of factors can influence the outcomes of consultation; several are discussed below.

Accountability

Today teachers are accountable for many student-related activities. They are accountable for how well the student responds to his/her educational program. They are expected to provide research-supported practices for all students. And they are expected to be able to provide data on how well students are achieving their educational objectives. Accountability of the outcomes of instructional practices is reflected in federal law and state standards. Because teachers have numerous responsibilities, it is important to acknowledge with the teacher the pressure in meeting all of these expectations. Helping the teacher to understand that the outcomes of the consultation is a shared responsibility between the consultant and the teacher is important. However, ultimately, the teacher is the primary professional responsible for the student's educational program. A goal of consultation, then, is to communicate to the teacher that the outcomes of the COMPASS consultation are consistent with the teacher's goal for the student—which is increased responsiveness of students to their educational programs.

Assessment

Standards vary state-by-state. States have academic content standards that emphasize areas of learning and achievement. Teachers have to be knowledgeable of portfolio assessment and alternative assessment strategies. In the spring, teachers may
change focus from IEP objectives to skills related to portfolio or alternate assessment. Often, the skills targeted in these assessments do not correspond to the objectives or skills targeted by the IEP. It is helpful to discuss this with the teacher and
help her or him see the link between IEP objectives and state academic content
standards. Thus, a consultant needs to have knowledge of state standards in order to
assist the teacher in seeing the links.

Individual Education Programs

The Individual Education Program is the road map that puts into place the direction
and course to be taken for the student. It creates the foundation from which decisions
regarding assessment, teaching plans, and accommodations and modifications occur.
Given the high importance placed on IEPs, we were surprised to find little guidance
on working with teachers on IEPs as part of consultation. We did find, much to our
regret, that IEP quality was generally poor across states, districts, schools, and teachers (Ruble, McGrew, Dalrymple, & Jung, 2010b). This is important because we also
found that the quality of the IEP was associated with how well the children responded
to their educational program. Thus, it is important for consultants to review with
teachers the quality of the IEP (how measurable are the objectives; how clear are the
descriptions of present levels of performance; how clear are the environmental supports?). Chapter 5 covers IEPs in more detail, includes a checklist to consider when
reviewing IEPs with teachers, and provides a more comprehensive discussion of this
issue, as IEP quality is associated with student outcomes.

Time

Time has been acknowledged as a critical factor in school-based services and a major
issue influencing consultation outcomes. Acceptability research suggests that logisti-
cal issues such as time and administrative support influence teacher's perceptions
(Sheridan & Steck, 1995) and that administrators need information on the importance
of parent–teacher collaboration. The COMPASS consultation and teacher coaching
package takes into account the need to be sensitive to teacher time. Direct interactions
require about 3 h for the initial COMPASS consultation and 4–6 h for follow-up sessions that last about 1–1.5 h each, totaling a maximum of 9 h throughout the year. Data
from our study suggest that the intervention does not negatively interfere with teacher
time or cause stress. Some teachers still may be concerned about the amount of time
required to implement teaching plans, keep data and monitor progress, and complete

other forms. Thus, it is necessary to plan the consultation and coaching sessions taking into account teacher time constraints and fit within the schedule and the student's routines. Because we have conducted experimental research on the COMPASS consultation package, we have distilled the necessary elements of paperwork to maximize teacher involvement to the critical aspects of the intervention and minimize teacher involvement in those areas not related to outcome.

Role As Classroom Manager

In our research, something that became apparent from observing several classrooms was the teacher role in the classroom. Some classrooms have an equal number of adults to students, while other classrooms may have two adults and 20 students. Classrooms vary as much as the differences in students with autism. But some of the common elements observed are teaching assistants and therapists who may work with a student within the classroom or stay with a student throughout the day. As consultant, it is important to explore with the teacher his/her perception of his/her role in the classroom and how this perception may influence effectiveness. Teachers who are new to the profession may be intimidated by teaching assistants who are older than themselves or who have worked in classrooms for many years. The teacher's role should be one of manager—someone who teaches students and also oversees the teaching assistants and ensures that student IEP objectives are clearly communicated to all who work with the students and are being monitored systematically and continually. It is the teacher, after all, who is legally responsible for the IEP.

Teacher As Consultant/Collaborator

Special education teachers may be expected to be able to monitor IEP objectives in all school environments, including general education classrooms and other special areas. In addition, special education teachers are also expected to be able to collaborate with their peers, other classroom teachers, and therapists as well as transfer their own skill and knowledge to classroom teaching assistants. The ability to work well with general education teachers, classroom assistants, and special area teachers provides additional skills not necessarily associated with the ability to work directly with the student. Nevertheless, it is important to take into consideration the skills necessary to work with others because students with autism attend all types of classrooms, often have teaching assistants, and must have teaching plans that include plans for generalization as part of their IEP objectives. Generalization plans often include teaching the student to perform the skill in different environments, with different people, and with different cues. Nevertheless, on an individual level, we found that some teachers had difficulty implementing the teaching plans in classrooms outside of their own. It was unclear if this difficulty related to acceptability, skills, time, or other issues. For students with autism in general education classrooms, there appeared to be more difficulty with the

special education teacher implementing teaching plans when involvement or collaboration with another teacher was necessary. Thus, it is important for the consultant to
discuss with the teacher specific strategies to engage other teachers, therapists, and
assistants as early in the planning process as possible.

The consultant may also need to work with the teacher to convey the priority of
individualization of the IEP goals within the total school environment. School principals vary tremendously in their understanding of the education of special needs
students. The teacher often becomes an advocate for the student in obtaining accommodations in the halls, cafeteria, bus area, or playground. Some schools have strict
school-wide disciplinary or behavioral rules that apply to each and every student.
One school we examined required students to get "cards" for various infractions
that led to a consequence of losing minutes at recess the following day. For a young
student with autism, just receiving a card caused so much anxiety that the rest of the
day was a loss. The consultant and the teacher worked out an individualized plan
that would still help the student learn acceptable behavior but was based on positive
behavior supports that were not counterproductive to his learning.

Parent and Student Considerations

Another role of the consultant is to assist teachers with understanding the different roles
that parents and teachers hold regarding the student with autism. Teachers have knowledge of and responsibility for many students, often focus on student deficits or skills to
be learned, have limited one-on-one contact with the student, are motivated to use
research-supported practices, and have chosen to work with students with disabilities.

Parents, on the other hand, have different perspectives and experiences. They are
experts on their own child and hold a more comprehensive view of the whole child.
They are responsible for the child 24 h each day for their lifetime. Living harmoni-
ously with the child and family is a key motivator. Research suggests that parents of
students with autism experience more stress compared to parents of students with
other developmental disabilities. Unlike teachers who have chosen to work with
students with disabilities, parents did not choose to have a child with ASD.

Although the roles are different for teachers and parents, both are equally valid.
Parents, as part of COMPASS consultation, play a key part in helping school personnel understand the student's history, how certain behaviors may have developed, how
family members respond, what is important and relevant for the family, and what
supports are available to the family. Perhaps the most important role of the parent is
that the parent speaks for, and often in the place of the student, who may be voiceless,
literally. The student's perspective is presumably represented by everyone, but if the
student is not involved or not able to be involved, this responsibility falls most heav-
ily on the parents. The consultant and teacher share goals of empowering parents and
caregivers because they are the lifelong advocates for the student. Teachers who
work well and communicate clearly with all parents demonstrate awareness, knowledge, and respect for their input as well as sensitivity to cultural differences. This

Table 4.1 Questions to consider prior to consultation

- What are consultation and coaching outcomes trying to achieve for the teacher, the student, and others?
- How will you measure progress toward the outcome(s)?
- How will you plan to monitor progress with the teacher using the measurement system?
- Are you an external or internal consultant, and have you thought about the implications?
- If you are internal, how will you
  - Address role clarity with the teacher and with administrators?
  - Discuss expectations of consultation and how it will terminate?
  - Discuss issues of confidentiality with the teacher?
- How will you assure the teacher that you are not evaluating her/him or sharing information with superiors?
- How will you assure that you are taking into account a culturally sensitive approach?

facilitates positive and satisfying partnerships. It also assists with generalization of student skills across environments and more consistent teaching approaches.

Student Characteristics

Much research has been completed on the characteristics of children with autism and how these characteristics relate to treatment outcomes. Intelligence, language, social abilities, and autism severity have been found to be associated with how well children respond to early intervention. Our preliminary research suggests that most student characteristics did not predict educational outcomes above and beyond the impact of the COMPASS intervention. This makes sense because COMPASS interventions are designed to be personalized to the student. The identification of teaching objectives and teaching strategies takes into account the student's present levels of performance, personal and environmental strengths and challenges, and parent and teacher concerns. We did find, however, that IQ predicted student outcomes and that more work needs to be done in implementing effective intervention strategies.

As students with autism are diverse, so are families. Particular attention to differences between the experiences and values of the consultant and those that may be a result of culture, ethnicity, race, economic and educational background differences in families must be given.

In summary, the ability to provide effective consultation and coaching is difficult. Multiple factors affect consultation. Some of the influences are under the control of the consultant, but many are not. It is the job of the consultant to be aware of all the various factors and use this knowledge continuously in evaluating progress toward outcomes. Questions to consider prior to beginning a consultation and coaching relationship with a teacher are provided in Table 4.1. Without clear outcomes at the start, it will be nearly impossible to monitor all the factors. But with authentic, open communication between the teacher and consultant combined with clearly stated goals that are observable and measurable, significant progress can result on behalf of the student.

Chapter 5
Writing Effective Individual Education Programs

Overview: This chapter provides more details that assist with the activities that are described in Chaps. 7 and 8. The consultant facilitates the consultation by guiding the participants in using all the available information about the student to select objectives in communication, social, and work skills. Objectives must be well written using suggestions provided in this chapter.

In this chapter we describe the following:

1. Best practices in educating students with autism using the National Research Council (NRC) recommendations and the Individuals with Disabilities Education Act mandates
2. How to write good IEP objectives
3. How to apply the concepts of maintenance and generalization of skills and include activities that address these concepts in a teaching plan
4. How to use an IEP checklist
5. Various ways to use the IEP checklist

According to the Individuals with Disabilities Education Act (IDEA), autism is defined as a developmental disability that significantly affects verbal and nonverbal communication and social interaction, is generally evident before age 3, and adversely affects a student's educational performance. Other characteristics associated with autism are engagement in repetitive activities and stereotyped movements, resistance to environmental change or change in daily routines, and unusual responses to sensory experiences (American Psychiatric Association, 2004).

Although students with autism share the label, they vary from one another according to intellectual ability (Chakrabarti & Fombonne, 2005; Jonsdottir et al., 2007), communication and social interaction skills (Castelloe & Dawson, 1993; O'Brien, 1996; Prizant & Wetherby, 2005; Wing & Gould, 1979), and other developmental domains (Beglinger & Smith, 2001) such as fine and gross motor skills, academic skills, and sensory processing abilities. Further, the characteristics of autism tend to change with age (Lord & Risi, 1998). Children, who were nonverbal at age 4, for example, may be verbal at age 10, but still not be able to engage in

L.A. Ruble et al., *Collaborative Model for Promoting Competence and Success for Students with ASD*, DOI 10.1007/978-1-4614-2332-4_5, © Springer Science+Business Media, LLC 2012

reciprocal conversation. Children who could not imitate the action of others at age 3 may be able to play with objects appropriately at age 7, but not cooperatively with other children. Although the core impairments of autism—social and communication skills—are shared across all children with the diagnosis, due to the unique blend of strengths and weaknesses of students with autism, teachers must tailor educational interventions to individual students rather than rely on the label to guide individual program development (Ruble & Dalrymple, 2002; Ruble, McGrew, Dalrymple & Jung 2010b).

To facilitate individualization of educational programs, schools are required to follow the mandates of IDEA that each student with a disability receives an Individual Education Plan (IEP) (USDOE, 2004). The IEP is the keystone of a successful program and has several goals. First, it puts in writing a commitment of resources to the student. Second, it serves as a management tool to ensure the identification of specialized interventions and need for ancillary services such as speech and language therapy and occupational therapy. Third, the IEP is a compliance and monitoring tool and acts as an evaluation device that facilitates measurement of student progress (Armenta & Beckers, 2006). Fourth, the IEP process mandates regular and systematic reviews of progress in order to promote general education curriculum participation (Burns, 2001). Fifth, IEPs can also be used to evaluate educational progress by providing a description of short-term objectives that lead to the attainment of larger and more comprehensive goal attainment (Rodger, 1995). Finally, IEPs provide a direct connection between teaching objectives and classroom activities that are evident and observable (Smith, Slattery, & Knopp, 1993). If IEP objectives are written specifically enough for observational coding, then data can be utilized to evaluate the success of intervention methods within the school setting. If it is determined that the student is not making progress toward the short-term objective (usually lasting one grading period), then the intervention can be changed without losing an entire year on a plan that is not working (Smith et al., 1993).

Best Practices

NRC Recommendations

According to the NRC, at a minimum, educational programs of students with autism should target social skills, communication, developmentally appropriate tasks/play activities that include a motivation system, fine and gross motor skills for age-appropriate activities, cognitive and academic skills, replacement skills for problematic behaviors, and organization skills that underlie success in a general education classroom. In essence, the NRC (2001) recommends comprehensive IEPs that target a range of social/communicative, adaptive, functional, academic, and cognitive abilities. These areas for IEP planning are summarized in the forms section in Chap. 7 (Overview of Best Practices for Individualized Education Plans (IEP) for Young Students with ASD).

Federal Law

Examples of required elements in the IEP as mandated by IDEA (2004) include a description of (a) the student's present levels of academic achievement and functional performance, (b) measurable goals that include benchmarks or short-term objectives for students who take alternate assessments based on alternate achievement standards, (c) measurement of student progress, (d) related services, and (e) program modifications and supports for school personnel.

Writing Good IEP Objectives

One of the biggest challenges for teachers of students with ASD (and for other students too) is writing social and communication skills objectives that are measurable and clear to the outside observer. See Table 5.1 for examples. IDEA (2004) stipulates that the IEP must include benchmarks or short-term objectives in the IEP for students who are on the alternate assessment route based on alternate assessment standards. We would expect that all students with ASD (there may be some notable exceptions) have IEP goals that are broken down into benchmarks or short-term objectives. Essential features of well-developed objectives include the following:

- Has a description of intermediate steps that indicate how progress toward meeting the annual goal will be measured.
- Is able to be attained within a year (target dates can be less than a year, such as by quarter or semester).
- Has identified the specific behaviors to be performed, criteria for attainment, evaluation/measurement procedures, and timelines for progress measurement (more detail on these features is below).
- Is sequenced developmentally (e.g., play with five toys in a functional manner; play with five toys using pretend play), incrementally (complete an independent work task within 5 min; complete two independent work tasks within 20 min), or by level of proficiency (e.g., from 25 to 50%; five out of eight opportunities).

Table 5.2 provides more details on the components of a well-developed IEP objective (Fig. 5.1).

Table 5.1 Examples of IEP objectives

During free play when offered a toy from a peer, Johnny will respond by taking the toy three times a day over 3 consecutive days

During independent work time with visual cues only, Amy will start and complete a familiar activity, such as matching, sorting, or categorizing items, two times a day for 5 of out 5 days

During breakfast, lunch, and snack time, Joey will initiate at least one request for a desired food using pictures three times a day for 8 out of 10 days

During structured play with a peer and verbal cues from the peer, Devon will imitate an action with an object two times a day over 4 consecutive days

Table 5.2 Components of a well-developed IEP objective

Component	Definition	Examples
Condition	The circumstances or setting when behavior is to be performed; this also includes the level of prompting that may be used (physical, verbal, gestural, verbal) from the adult or peer; when prompts are not listed, it is assumed the skill is to be performed independently by the student	Given a structured small group of 2–3 students Given familiar 1–2 step directions (list to be provided) During snack/lunch time when given one verbal cue (e.g., What do you want?) Given two different situations where he/she needs help and has a visual cue (to be identified) and adult is within 2 ft. During a structured playtime with a social, verbal peer and with peer prompts only and with familiar toys During a work session and with a familiar work task that can be done independently
Performance	The action or behavior the student is to do	Follow familiar directions Point to an object Verbalize a want/need Complete familiar work task Initiate request toward peer Make on topic comments Provide full sentence answers
Criterion	The standard of performance of the behavior	8 out of 10 opportunities 5 different objects, 5 times each over 5 play times 3 tasks each for 10 times Each day of the week 10 consecutive times
Measurement	The procedures for evaluating progress toward the objective	Direct observation of skill Videotape review Products (homework, written assignments) Parent/teacher report Tests Checklists
Time line	The time line for determining progress toward objectives	Annual: Biannual Quarterly: Daily Semester: Weekly

Condition	Performance	Criteria
Measurement	Time Line	

Fig. 5.1 Template for writing a well-developed IEP objective

Maintenance and Generalization

Maintenance and generalization refer to what happens when the teaching plan is stopped or when the student is in a different classroom, home or the community, working with different teachers, using different materials, or interacting with different peers. Without plans in place, the student may lose the skills that he once learned. Helping the student maintain the skills once the specific teaching plan is no longer in place is a necessity. Further, developing specific teaching plans that include teaching the student to transfer the skills to another situation is necessary. For students with ASD, generalization does not happen without intention and specific teaching.

COMPASS consultation is designed with generalization in mind. At the outset, teaching objectives are identified with parent and teacher input so that important skills that have meaning for home and school are targeted. Also included is the development of specific teaching plans that are shared with parents. Still, this is not enough to ensure maintenance and generalization. Other suggestions from Zirpoli and Melloy (1993) are:

1. Teach skills in natural settings
2. Share teaching plans with other adults and caregivers
3. Implement teaching plans in a variety of settings
4. Use natural reinforcers; if a reinforcer such as food is being used, fade to more natural consequences
5. Shift from continuous reinforcement to intermittent reinforcement
6. Gradually shift from immediate reinforcement to delays in reinforcement in the natural environment
7. Reinforce when you see the student display behavior in untrained settings or generalized activities
8. Focus on behaviors that will be reinforced by others
9. Ensure that the skill is within the student's skill set before working on generalization
10. Utilize environmental supports that will facilitate the occurrence of skills

IEP Evaluation Checklist

To assist with the development of a high quality IEP, we have provided an IEP Evaluation Checklist. This checklist was used in a study to evaluate the strengths and weaknesses of IEPs and to provide recommendations for improving IEPs (Ruble et al., 2010b). Our research showed that students with IEPs that contained objectives that were more sensitive to the needs of students with autism (i.e., IEPs that had social, communication, and work/learning skill objectives) and were more measurable made more progress on their selected objectives at the end of the school year.

Ways to Use the Checklist

There are many ways the IEP checklist can be used. The first purpose is for conducting a review of the quality of current IEPs. The IEP checklist can be used to identify weaknesses in the IEP, such as a lack of measurable objectives or a lack of social skills, communication, or learning skills objectives. The identification of weaknesses can be used as a way to establish goals for COMPASS consultation, in-service training, and other professional development efforts to improve IEPs.

A second purpose of the IEP checklist is to monitor the effects of COMPASS consultation. Recall in Chap. 4 the COMPASS Mediation Model tested. We have provided it again here (Fig. 5.2).

In the discussion of this model, we reported the results of two elements that act as active ingredients of COMPASS consultation. One of the elements was IEP quality. We expect COMPASS to result in better IEPs because the consultation ensures that (a) objectives sensitive to the needs of students with autism and described by the NRC (2001) are included in the IEP and (b) the objectives targeted as a result of COMPASS consultation are measurable and added to the IEP. The questions in the IEP checklist that have an asterisk beside them are the areas we expect to change as a result of COMPASS consultation. The other questions are also important but are not expected to change as a result of COMPASS consultation. Thus, the tool can be used to measure IEP quality before and after COMPASS to ensure that those who receive COMPASS are making changes to the IEP.

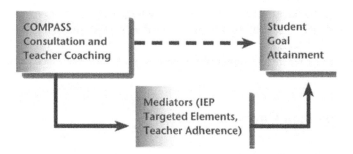

Fig. 5.2 COMPASS mediation model tested

Appendix IEP Evaluation Form

Student's Name:_____ DOB/Age:_____

Reviewer's Name:_____ Date of IEP:_____

Instructions: The evaluation form has two major parts: A and B. Part A has two components. The first section evaluates the descriptions of the present levels of performance. The second section addresses the IEP as a whole.

Part B is concerned with specific goals or objectives. The goal is the broad domain; the objective is the specific skill that is targeted under the goal. It is recommended that the entire IEP be reviewed before it is scored.

Part A: Analysis of Overall IEP

Directions: Determine if the following education performance areas are described as an area of need (if the area is checked, but no description is provided, mark "no"; if any kind of description is provided, mark "yes").

Area	No	Yes
1. Communication status		
2. Academic performance		
3. Health, vision, hearing, motor abilities		
4. Social and emotional status		
5. General intelligence (cognitive)		
6. Overall quality of description of student's performance relative to the general curriculum or developmental status is clear enough to establish well-written goals for the student. Code "no" if there is no reference to grade, age, or developmental equivalents/performance.		

Comments:

Review of Related Services

Instructions: If related services are provided, indicate "yes" and the amount of time the service is provided per week.

	No	Yes	Time of week
7. Speech therapy			
8. Occupational therapy			
9. Physical therapy			
10. Other:			

Instructions: Review the overall IEP and determine to what degree each indicator is provided. Use the Likert scale that ranges from 0 ("no/not at all") to 2 ("very much/ clearly evident"). "Not applicable" is NA. Examples of IEP objectives for each of these indicators follows the checklist.

	0	1	2
	No/not at all		Very much/ clearly evident

Indicator (examples of the IEP objectives for items 13–20 are provided at the end of this IEP Evaluation Form)	NA	0	1	2
11. Annual goals include goals from the COMPASS consultation				
12. Parental concerns are described (code "2" if *any* concerns are listed)				
13. Includes goals/objectives for social skills to improve involvement in school and family activities (i.e., social objective is targeted for improved functioning in school/or family life). Must have more than 1 objective to code "2" ***				
14. Includes goals/objectives for expressive, receptive, and nonverbal communication skills (code "NA" if *communication* is not listed as an area of need in present levels of performance, code "0" if communication is listed as area of need but there are no communication goals/objectives, code "1" if there is only one goal for receptive and expressive language, code "2" if there are goals for both receptive and expressive language). ***				
15. Includes goals/objectives for symbolic functional communication system (PECS, assistive technology, etc). Code as "NA" if student shows evidence of conversational speech in the present levels of performance. When augmentative/alternative communication (ACC) isn't an objective but listed as a support for objectives, code as "1." ***				
16. Includes goals/objectives for engagement in tasks or play that are developmentally appropriate (must emphasize a focus on developmental skills such as attending, sitting in circle, taking turns, etc., rather than academic), including an appropriate motivational system (code "1" if developmentally appropriate but no motivation system is described).				
17. Includes goals/objectives for fine and gross motor skills to be utilized when engaging in age appropriate activities. Must have more than one objective to code "2."				

(continued)

0	1	2
No/not at all		Very much/ clearly evident

(continued)

	NA	0	1	2
18. Includes goals/objectives for basic cognitive and academic thinking skills (sorting, letters, numbers, reading, etc). Must have more than one objective to code "2."				
19. Includes goals/objectives for replacement of problem behaviors with appropriate behaviors (evidence is provided that the skill is designed to replace a problem behavior). Must have more than one objective to code "2."				
20. Includes goals/objectives for organizational skills and other behaviors that underlie success in a general education classroom (independently completing a task, following instructions, asking for help, etc). Must have more than one objective to code "2." ***				
21. Objectives are individualized and adapted from the state academic content standards (i.e., goals are assumed to be the academic content standard). Code "2" if most are individualized but some are not; code "1" if some are individualized, but most are not.				

*** Denotes targeted indicators that are expected to change as a result of COMPASS consultation.

22. Number of goals in the IEP: _____

23. Number of objectives in the IEP: _____

24. Is the need for extended school year addressed?   □ Yes   □ No

25. Is extended school year recommended as a service?   □ Yes   □ No   □ Not Addressed

Part B: Analysis of Specific IEP Objectives

Note: Use with COMPASS objectives and/or with as many objectives as desired

Objective: _____

_____

IEP goal No. and page No. on the IEP:_____ No. of objectives under goal:_____

Objective Code (select from options below):_____

0 = Academic; 1 = Social; 2 = Communication; 3 = Learning/Work Skills; 4 = Motor/Sensory; 5=Self-help; 6=Behavior

Instructions: Code each objective (not goal). Use the following Likert scale that ranges from 0 ("no/not at all") to 2 ("very much/clearly evident"). "Not applicable" is NA

0	1	2
No/not at all		Very much/ clearly evident

Indicator	NA	0	1	2
26. The student's present level of performance is described for this objective (don't rate quality here). If a simple description like one sentence is given, code "2."				
27. The student's performance of this objective (in summary of present levels of performance) is described in a manner that links it *specifically* to the **general** curriculum.				
28. The student's performance of this objective (in summary of present levels of performance) is described in a manner that links it *specifically* to **developmental** curriculum.				
29. This objective is able to be measured in behavioral terms. Code "1" if it can be observed, code "2" if the description of target behavior is clear for proper measurement of goal achievement through observation.***				
30. The conditions under which the behavior is to occur are provided, i.e., when, where, with whom.***				
31. The criterion for goal acquisition is described, i.e., rate, frequency, percentage, latency, duration, as well as a timeline for goal attainment is described specifically for objective (other than for length of IEP).***				
32. A method of goal measurement is described. Code "1" if method of measurement is just checked according to a preset list and not individualized specific to objective.				
33. Is Specially Designed Instruction individualized to the objective? (Code "0" if there is no SDI specified, code "1" if SDI is checked off but not specifically designed for that objective, code "2" for individualized SDI).				

Note: Item with *** is a targeted indicator expected to change as a result of COMPASS consultation.

Examples of IEP Objectives for Each Indicator Described in Part A

Indicator Item 6

Example: During a 10-min free play activity and with a verbal or visual cue, will provide eye contact to adult/peer partner at least three times during the activity within 6 weeks.

Example: When participating in a social skills group with teachers and/or peers, will have two or more verbal exchanges three out of four times for each session for three consecutive sessions as observed and recorded in monitoring data by teachers and/ or staff by the end of the school year.

Indicator Item 7

Example (Receptive Communication): When presented with an object or picture and the question "Do you want____," he will verbally answer yes or no with a visual prompt and accept his answer 4 out of 5 times over 4 consecutive days.

Example (Receptive Communication): When an adult is within 6 feet and says child's name, child will turn and look toward the speaker with no more than 2 verbal cues, 3 out of 4 trials a day for 3 consecutive days by the end of the grading period.

Example (Expressive/Receptive Communication): During a structured activity, will engage in three conversational exchanges on a topic with one peer using an appropriate voice level with visual and/or peer cues for 4 of 5 consecutive sessions by the end of the school year

Indicator Item 8

Example of a Score of 2: During free play, breakfast, lunch and work time, will request 10 items/activities/food choices through picture exchange or voice output at least one time for each of 4 daily activities over 3 consecutive days by the end of the school year.

Example of a Score of 2: Given a structured "lesson," student will give a picture to an adult to indicate something he wants for 3 objects/foods with 2 physical prompts, 4 out of 5 times over 2 consecutive weeks for each.

Example of a Code of 1: During free play and when given three choices, will make a preferred choice on three out of four trials at least once daily for 3 consecutive days in 6 weeks. (Picture exchange listed in specially designed instruction for this objective).

Indicator Item 9

Example: Given structured play time, will imitate three different adult/child actions with at least five different objects twice a day for each object for 4 out of 5 days within 12 weeks.

Example: When given familiar tasks in structured work time, will finish 3 tasks with 1 environmental cue to start and with an adult 3 feet away, with no more than 1 redirection (gestural, verbal) 2 times a day for 5 consecutive days in 36 weeks.

Indicator Item 10

Example: During written activities and a model, will hold a writing utensil using a tripod grasp at least 80% of the time during a 10-min activity daily for four consecutive days by 12 weeks.

Example: During work time and with peer models, will cut out three different forms including curvy and/or wavy lines staying within 1/2 in. of the lines at least 8 out of 10 trials 3 out of 4 days in 36 weeks.

Indicator Item 11

Example: During math, when given a visual example and a verbal prompt to start, will complete 10, 2 digit addition and subtraction problems with regrouping with 80% accuracy for 3 consecutive days by 18 weeks.

Example: During reading group, will read and demonstrate understanding of 12 new words each week in 36 weeks.

Indicator Item 12

Example: When denied a request and offered an alternative, will accept the alternative with reduced physical aggression (from baseline) with no more than 50% aggressive acts (from baseline) per day across 2 weeks by the end of the school year.

Example: Will follow a relaxation routine with two verbal cues/visual cues and be able to continue in the current activity or setting without escalating behaviors (whining, yelling out) on five consecutive occasions when he is starting to be upset/ anxious within 12 weeks.

Indicator Item 13

Example: During a structured work activity when student needs help, will verbally ask adult/peer with a visual cue, "Help me please" 4 of 5×a day during a 2-week period by the end of the school year.

Example: Given a teacher directed lesson, the student will raise his hand, wait to be called on, and give his response to a teacher question with visual cues for four of five consecutive sessions.

Chapter 6
COMPASS Consultation Action Plan: Step A

Overview: This chapter covers Step A of the COMPASS Consultation Action Plan, which is conducted prior to the consultation. This information will inform the framework for the student's personalized COMPASS profile.

In this chapter, we describe Step A, the first of two procedural steps, of a COMPASS Consultation Action Plan. This includes:

1. Gathering information about the student from consultant observations and from the caregiver and teacher reports using the COMPASS Challenges and Supports Form for Caregivers and Teachers.
2. Completing the COMPASS Challenges and Supports Joint Summary Form (JSF).

There are a total of two steps to the COMPASS Consultation Action Plan that help the consultant prepare for the collaborative consultation (see Table 6.1). In Step A, which is explained in this chapter, the consultant gathers current information about the student from teachers and caregivers before the consultation begins. Then, in Step B, which is outlined in Chap. 7, the information gathered in the first step is shared, giving all participants a common understanding of the student's current personal and environmental challenges and the personal and environmental supports necessary for success. Then, the consultant, caregiver, and teacher prioritize goals, write measurable objectives, and develop the teaching plan and identify environmental supports for each objective. Forms and handouts that represent Steps A and B of the action plan are provided at the end of these two chapters.

Subsequent to COMPASS consultation is teacher coaching. These procedures are discussed in Chap. 8—Coaching Sessions: Implementing Plans and Monitoring Progress.

L.A. Ruble et al., *Collaborative Model for Promoting Competence and Success for Students with ASD*, DOI 10.1007/978-1-4614-2332-4_6, © Springer Science+Business Media, LLC 2012

Table 6.1 COMPASS consultation action plan for students with autism

Step A—activities prior to a COMPASS consultation (Chap. 6)

Gather information about the student from consultant observations and from the caregiver and teacher reports using the COMPASS challenges and supports form for caregivers and teachers

Complete COMPASS challenges and supports joint summary form

Step B—activities during a COMPASS consultation (Chap. 7)

Discuss COMPASS consultation training packet

Discuss COMPASS consultation joint summary

Identify and come to consensus on three prioritized objectives and write measurable objectives

Develop COMPASS teaching plans for each measurable objective

Step A: Activities Conducted Prior to a COMPASS Consultation

The primary activity in this chapter sets the stage for developing the educational foundation for the student and is the first step described in the COMPASS Consultation Action Plan for Students with Autism. Step A helps the consultant prepare for the collaborative consultation by providing forms especially developed for students with ASD for completion by caregivers and teachers so that current information is gathered about the student.

There are two parts to Step A:

Gather Information About the Student Using COMPASS Challenges and Supports Form for Caregivers and Teachers

Gathering information about the student can be completed in several ways, such as the consultant conducting a direct assessment and observation and the consultant obtaining information from teachers and caregivers using rating scales and questionnaires.

Consultant Observations

The assessment process to obtain consultation observations includes required activities and recommended activities. Although we recommend that the functional assessment include the consultant having direct interactions with the student, it may not always be feasible to conduct an observation or evaluation of the student prior to consultation. Therefore, information can also be gathered from parents/caregivers, teachers, therapists, record review, observations, and other means such as videotape review. In our earlier consultation work, we asked teachers and caregivers to videotape the student during structured and unstructured activities at school (and home if possible) that depicted the student's typical communication, social, and learning skills. Although this was very helpful, an obvious pitfall was that it did not allow us to interact with the student directly.

Necessary consultant assessment activities include the following:

- Review of previous medical, psychological, language, and other assessment reports.
- Review the current IEP for social, communication, and learning skill objectives and measurability of objectives (see Chap. 5 for more information on IEPs).
- Review videotapes or conduct observations of the student during a structured work activity in the classroom or with the consultant.
- Review videotapes or conduct observations of the student during unstructured activities, such as free play, recess, and lunch.

Consultant assessment activities that are not necessary but are recommended include:

- Conduct a direct assessment of the student's developmental, adaptive behavior, and cognitive skills using standardized measures.
- Conduct direct assessment of the student's social, communication, and learning skills from criterion-referenced measures or observation.

A *Consultant Assessment Checklist* is provided in the forms section at the end of the chapter, which can help facilitate the collection of the consultant observations. In our research, we have found that direct student interactions are valuable because they allow the consultant not only to conduct his or her own functional assessment of the student's cognitive, problem solving, social, language, and learning skills, but also to examine how the student responds using various environmental supports. For example, during the assessment, the consultant can use a work-reward routine and a visual schedule. It is helpful to know if the student understands the use of visuals for these purposes and whether student engagement and motivation during assessment can be enhanced. The consultant can also set up the assessment to elicit certain learning skills (see item 8, "Learning Skills," in the COMPASS Challenges and Supports Form for Caregivers and Teachers) to record how well the student understands and demonstrates starting a work task, finishing a work task, asking for help, etc.

Caregiver and Teacher Reports

To help gather information that is representative of the student at home, in the community, and at school, the consultant will present the *COMPASS Challenges and Supports Form for Caregivers and Teachers* to the caregiver and the teacher to fill out separately. This form asks the caregiver and the teacher to indicate the child's adaptive skills, problem behaviors, social and play skills, communication skills, sensory challenges, sensory supports, learning skills, environmental challenges and supports, and to list concerns that interfere with the child's success. Family members complete one set, and the student's primary special education teacher completes a set. If the student is in a general education classroom, receives speech and language therapy or occupational therapy, or receives instruction from other school personnel, it is recommended that their input be sought and added. For example, the occupational therapist can provide information on the student's fine and gross motor skills and sensory issues. The speech language pathologist has information regarding the student's communication strengths and weaknesses and pragmatic difficulties that can be shared.

Complete COMPASS Challenges and Supports Joint Summary Form

Once the parent/caregiver and teacher complete their sets of the COMPASS Challenges and Support Form for Caregivers and Teachers and return them to the consultant prior to the consultation, the consultant then summarizes the information in a *COMPASS Challenges and Support Joint Summary Form*. At the first consultation (Step B), the consultant will provide this summary to the caregivers and teachers. This summary organizes the information and also ensures that all participants have a common understanding of the student's personal and environmental challenges, as well as the student's personal and environmental strengths.

Directions on completing the three COMPASS forms discussed in this chapter are provided with the forms.

Appendix A   Consultant Assessment Checklist

It is necessary for the consultant to obtain information directly or indirectly about the child. Activities that are necessary and those that are recommended but not required are as follows:

Necessary Activities

A. Gather most recent assessment information and provide the following details:

Area evaluated	Date of evaluation	Findings
Medical		
Psychological		
Receptive and expressive language		
Fine and gross motor		
Adaptive behavior		

B. Review current IEP for social, communication, and learning skill objectives and measurability of objectives (see Chap. 8 for more information on IEPs).

Domain	IEP objective
Social	
Communication	
Learning skills	
Other	

C. Review videotape or conduct observation of student during a structured work activity in the classroom or with the consultant, observe how the student initiates and responds, communicates, and works independently.

Activity	Description and length	Observations

D. Review videotape or conduct observation of the student during unstructured activities, such as free play, recess, and lunch and observe how the student initiates and responds, communicates with adults and peers and how they respond to him/her.

Activity	Description and length	Observations

Recommended But Not Required

A. Conduct direct assessment of child's developmental, adaptive behavior, and cognitive skills using standardized measures.

Assessment tool	Skills evaluated	Results and observations

B. Conduct direct assessment of child's social, communication, and learning skills from criterion-referenced measures or observation.

Assessment tool	Skills evaluated	Results and observations

Appendix B   COMPASS Challenges and Supports Form for Caregivers and Teachers/Service Providers

Child's/Student's Name: _____

Date: _____

Your Name: _____

Your Relationship to Child: _____

1. Likes, Strengths, Frustrations and Fears

The information you provide is vital in understanding how to build a competency model for your child/student.

Directions: Please list all the activities, objects, events, people, food, topics, or anything that is preferred by your child/student. These help identify ways to motivate and skills on which to build.

Likes/Preferences/Interests:	Comments:

Strengths or Abilities:	Comments:

Directions: Please list and describe the fears and frustrations of your child/student. Please be specific about the situations in which these occur and the behavior your child/student shows.

Frustrations: **Comments:**

Fears: **Comments:**

2. Adaptive Skills

Directions: Please answer each item using the scale as it presently applies to your child/student, with "1" meaning "not at all a problem" and "4" meaning "very much a problem." Add examples and notes as desired.

	Not at all			Very much
Self-management				
Performing basic self-care independently (such as toileting, dressing, eating, using utensils)	1	2	3	4
Entertaining self in free time	1	2	3	4
Changing activities—transitioning	1	2	3	4
Sleeping	1	2	3	4
Responding to others				
Following 1 or 2 step direction	1	2	3	4
Accepting "no"	1	2	3	4
Answering questions	1	2	3	4
Accepting help	1	2	3	4
Accepting correction	1	2	3	4
Being quiet when required	1	2	3	4
Understanding group behaviors				
Coming when called to group	1	2	3	4
Staying within certain places—lines, circles, chairs, desks	1	2	3	4
Participating with the group	1	2	3	4
Talking one at a time	1	2	3	4
Picking up, cleaning up, straightening up, putting away	1	2	3	4
Understanding community expectations				
Understanding who is a stranger	1	2	3	4
Going to places in the community (place of worship, stores, restaurants, malls, homes)	1	2	3	4
Understanding safety (such as streets, seat belts)	1	2	3	4
Managing transportation (Cars/buses)	1	2	3	4

3. Problem Behaviors*

Directions: Please answer each item on the scale of 1–4 as it presently applies to your child/student, with "1" meaning "not at all a problem" and "4" meaning "very much a problem."

		Not at all			Very much
1.	Acting impulsively, without thinking	1	2	3	4
2.	Hitting or hurting others	1	2	3	4
3.	Damaging or breaking things that belong to others	1	2	3	4
4.	Screaming or yelling	1	2	3	4
5.	Having sudden mood changes	1	2	3	4
6.	Having temper tantrums	1	2	3	4
7.	Having a low frustration tolerance; becoming easily angered or upset	1	2	3	4
8.	Crying easily	1	2	3	4
9.	Being overly quiet, shy, or withdrawn	1	2	3	4
10.	Acting sulky or sad	1	2	3	4
11.	Being underactive or lacking in energy	1	2	3	4
12.	Engaging in behaviors that may be distasteful to others, such as nose-picking or spitting	1	2	3	4
13.	Touching him/herself inappropriately	1	2	3	4
14.	Engaging in compulsive behaviors; repeating certain acts over and over	1	2	3	4
15.	Hitting or hurting him/herself	1	2	3	4
16.	Becoming overly upset when others touch or move his/her belongings	1	2	3	4
17.	Laughing/giggling at inappropriate times	1	2	3	4
18.	Ignoring or walking away from others during interactions or play	1	2	3	4
19.	Touching others inappropriately	1	2	3	4
20.	Engaging in unusual mannerisms such as hand-flapping or spinning	1	2	3	4
21.	Having to play or do things in the same exact way each time	1	2	3	4
22	Having difficulty calming him/herself down when upset or excited	1	2	3	4
23.	Other: _____	1	2	3	4

*Items are based on the Triad Social Skills Assessment
Add comments:

4. Social and Play Skills

Directions: Please rate the following statements on a scale of 1–4, with 1 meaning "not very well" and 4 meaning "very well." Please answer each question first in terms of the child's interactions with adults, and then with children.

How well does the child/student	With adults				With children			
	Not Very well			Very well	Not Very well			Very well
Social awareness								
1. Look toward a person who is talking to him/her	1	2	3	4	1	2	3	4
2. Accept others being close to him/her	1	2	3	4	1	2	3	4
3. Watch people for extended periods of time	1	2	3	4	1	2	3	4
4. Respond to another person's approach by smiling or vocalizing	1	2	3	4	1	2	3	4
5. Initiate interactions for social reasons	1	2	3	4	1	2	3	4
Joint attention skills								
6. Look at something another person points to	1	2	3	4	1	2	3	4
7. Show something to a person and look for person's reaction	1	2	3	4	1	2	3	4
8. Point at an object or event to direct another person's attention to share enjoyment	1	2	3	4	1	2	3	4
9. Share smile by looking back and forth between object and person	1	2	3	4	1	2	3	4
Imitation								
10. Imitate sounds another person makes	1	2	3	4	1	2	3	4
11. Imitate what another person does with an object (such as a person makes toy airplane fly, the child repeats action)	1	2	3	4	1	2	3	4
12. Imitate body movements of others (such as clap when others clap, play Simon Says)	1	2	3	4	1	2	3	4
13. Imitate and expand upon other's actions with toys (such as peer beats drum, child beats drum and also starts to march)	1	2	3	4	1	2	3	4

(continued)

(continued)

How well does the child/student

Play	With adults				With children			
	Not Very well			Very well	Not Very well			Very well
14. Take turns within familiar routines (such as rolls a ball back and forth)	1	2	3	4	1	2	3	4
15. Share toys	1	2	3	4	1	2	3	4
16. Play interactively around a common theme	1	2	3	4	1	2	3	4
17. Repair breakdowns during interactions (such as the child repeats or changes own behavior when other person seems confused or ignores)	1	2	3	4	1	2	3	4
18. Pretends to do something or be something (such as that a plate is a hat by putting it on, to be a policeman, to have a tea party, that a doll is a teacher)	1	2	3	4	1	2	3	4

5. Communication Skills

Directions: Please describe how your child/student lets you know the following communicative messages through words or actions. Indicate any method your child/student uses to indicate the message. For example, if s/he does not use words, but instead takes you by the hand to request juice, you would write that he takes you by the hand. If your child/student uses words, write what s/he says; or if a combination of ways are used, describe all ways.

Making Requests
1. Food
2. Objects
3. An activity
4. To use the toilet
5. Attention
6. Help
7. To play
8. Information
9. A choice
Expressing Refusals
1. "Go away"
2. "No, I won't do it" or "I don't want it"
3. "I want to be finished" or "I want to stop doing this"
Expressing Thoughts
1. Greeting to others
2. Comments about people/environment
3. Confusion or "I don't know"
4. Comments about errors or things wrong
5. Asks about past or future events
6. Agreement

(continued)

(continued)

Expressing Feelings
1. Angry/mad/frustrated
2. Pain/illness/hurt
3. Happy/excited
4. Hurt feelings/upset
5. Afraid
6. Sad

6. Sensory Challenges

Directions: Please put a check before each statement that describes your child/student.

Sound/Auditory

- ☐ Has been diagnosed with hearing problem at some time
- ☐ Reacts to unexpected sounds
- ☐ Fears some noises
- ☐ Distracted by certain sounds
- ☐ Confused about direction of sounds
- ☐ Makes self-induced noises

- ☐ Fails to listen or pay attention to what is said to him/her
- ☐ Talks a great deal
- ☐ Own talking interferes with listening
- ☐ Overly sensitive to some sounds
- ☐ Seeks out certain noises or sounds
- ☐ Other:_____

Taste

- ☐ Has an eating problem
- ☐ Dislikes certain foods and textures
- ☐ Will only eat a small variety of foods
- ☐ Tastes/eats nonedibles

- ☐ Explores environment by tasting
- ☐ Puts most things in his/her mouth
- ☐ Constant chewing on something
- ☐ Other:_____

Sight/Vision

- ☐ Has trouble discriminating shapes, colors
- ☐ Is sensitive to light—squints, wants to wear hats or sunglasses
- ☐ Has trouble following with eyes
- ☐ Does not make much eye contact
- ☐ Is distracted by some/too much visual stimuli
- ☐ Becomes excited when confronted with a variety of visual stimuli
- ☐ Dislikes having eyes covered

- ☐ Excited by vistas and open spaces
- ☐ Hesitates going up or down stairs, curbs, or climbing equipment
- ☐ Upset by things looking different (spills, spots)
- ☐ Makes decisions about food, clothing, objects by sight
- ☐ Closely examines objects or hands
- ☐ Wants environment in certain order
- ☐ Other:_____

Touch/Tactile

- ☐ Has to know someone is going to touch ahead of time
- ☐ Dislikes being held or cuddled
- ☐ Seems irritated when touched or bumped by peers
- ☐ Explores environment by touching objects
- ☐ Dislikes the feel of certain clothing
- ☐ Refuses to touch certain things
- ☐ Over- or underdresses for the temperature or is unaware of temperature

- ☐ Does not like showers or rain on self
- ☐ Mouths objects or clothing
- ☐ Refuses to walk on certain surfaces
- ☐ Dislikes having hair, face, or mouth touched
- ☐ Upset by sticky, gooey hands
- ☐ Touches items with feet before hands
- ☐ Does not like to hold hands
- ☐ Pinches, bites, or hurts her- or himself

Smell/Olfactory

- □ Sensitive to smells
- □ Smells objects, food, people, toys more than usual
- □ Xplores environment by smelling
- □ Reacts defensively to some smells
- □ Ignores strong odors
- □ Seeks out certain odors
- □ Other:_____

Movement/Vestibular

- □ Seems fearful in space (teeter-totter, climbing)
- □ Arches back when held or moved
- □ Spins or whirls self around
- □ Moves parts of body a great deal
- □ Walks on toes
- □ Appears clumsy, bumping into things and falling
- □ Avoids balance activities
- □ Does not like to be around people in motion
- □ Bumps into things and/or people
- □ Other:_____

Visual/Perceptual Motor

- □ Has trouble with paper/pencil activities
- □ Has difficulty with time perception
- □ Has difficulty with body in space, moving appropriately
- □ Has problems with use of some tools
- □ Has problems organizing materials and moving them appropriately
- □ Is distracted by doors and cupboards being open, holes, or motion
- □ Other:_____

7. Sensory Supports

Directions: Please put a check next to the item that pertains to your child/student.

Sound/Auditory

- ☐ Likes music
- ☐ Likes to sing and/or dance

☐ Other: _____

Taste

- ☐ Has definite eating preferences

☐ Other: _____

Sight/Vision

- ☐ Enjoys watching moving things/ bright objects
- ☐ Enjoys patterns or shiny surfaces

☐ Likes TV, VCR, videos

☐ Likes the computer

☐ Other: _____

Touch/Tactile

- ☐ Likes to be touched
- ☐ Likes hugs and cuddling when he/she initiates it
- ☐ Likes to play in water
- ☐ Likes baths or swimming pools
- ☐ Seeks out mud, sand, clay to touch
- ☐ Prefers deep touching rather than soft

☐ Prefers certain textures of clothing

☐ Likes being rolled or sandwiched between blankets/cushions

☐ Likes rough and tumble play

☐ Other: _____

Movement/Vestibular

- ☐ Enjoys rocking, swinging, spinning
- ☐ Likes being tossed in the air
- ☐ Likes to run
- ☐ Likes and needs to move

☐ Likes to climb, seldom falls

☐ Other: _____

Visual/Perceptual Motor

- ☐ Relies on knowing location of furniture, stationary objects
- ☐ Likes to draw and reproduce figures

☐ Other:_____

8. Learning Skills*

Directions: Please answer each item on the scale of 1–4 as it presently applies to your child/student's level of independence, with "1" meaning "not at all" and "4" meaning "very much."

		Not at all			Very much
1.	Child clearly understands the end goal of an activity, recognizes what he/she must do to be finished, and persists on the task to completion	1	2	3	4
2.	Child realizes when he/she is running into difficulty and has some way of letting the adult know he/she needs help	1	2	3	4
3.	Once an activity is under way, the adult can walk away from the child and he/she will keep working until finished, maintaining at least fairly good attention to what he/she is doing	1	2	3	4
4.	Child finishes work and remembers on his/her own to let the adult know (e.g., by bringing work to adult, calling adult, raising his/her hand)	1	2	3	4
5.	Child looks forward to earning a reward, knows it's next, works toward it, may ask for it or go get it on his/her own when work is finished	1	2	3	4
6.	Child is able to wait briefly for a direction (anticipates that he/she is about to be asked to do something), is able to wait briefly for his/her turn with a toy (anticipating that it's about to return him/her), and / or wait for something to happen	1	2	3	4
7.	Child may be distracted by outside sights and sounds or inner distractions (evident perhaps in singing to him/herself, gazing off, lining up materials) but is able to refocus attention to work on his/her own after a short time and without a prompt or reminder from the adult	1	2	3	4
8.	When one activity is finished, child will look for another to complete	1	2	3	4
9.	Child can organize his/her responses to perform tasks when multiple materials are in front of him/her (e.g., a stack of cards for sorting)	1	2	3	4
10.	Child recognizes when one strategy is not working and tries another way	1	2	3	4
11.	Child recognizes his/her own mistakes and goes back and corrects them (e.g., takes little peg out of big hole to make room for correct peg)				

*From TRIAD, adapted from Division TEACCH

9. Environmental Challenges

Describe environmental challenges of the child/student. Environmental challenges are factors that interfere with the child's learning. Examples are loud or confusing environments, lack of communication system or lack of sociable peers.

☐ Behavioral/Knowledge/Attitude of Other People Variables (such as inability to communicate clearly to the student, teach skills necessary for the activity, establish positive work or play routines).

☐ Procedural/Organizational (such as noisy environments, lack of visual supports, lack of effective transition routines).

☐ Temporal (such as lack or ineffective use of visual supports to understand passage of time or when activity is finished).

□ Spatial (such as lack of personal space or clear boundaries).

10. Environmental Supports

Describe environmental supports of the child/student. Environmental supports are factors that facilitate learning. Examples are positive routines, use of rewards, and use of visuals supports.

☐ Behavioral/Knowledge/Attitude of Other People Variables (such as is able to communicate clearly to the student, teach skills necessary for the activity, establish positive work or play routines).

☐ Procedural/Organizational (such as uncluttered environments, visual supports for understanding work routines, positive transition routines).

☐ Temporal (such as visual supports to understand passage of time or when activity is finished).

□ Spatial (such as personal space to work and calm down, clear boundaries).

11. Summary of Concerns

Directions: Please list one or two concerns under each area that you have about your child/student as they pertain to succeeding at home and school and being a competent person.

Social and Play Skills

1.
2.

Communication Skills

1.
2.

Learning Skills

1.
2.

Adaptive Skills

1.
2.

List any others on the back of this page.

Appendix C   Instructions for Completing COMPASS Challenges and Supports Joint Summary Form

In this section, we provide the COMPASS Challenges and Supports JSF. Using this form, you will summarize the information provided by the COMPASS Challenges and Supports Form for Caregivers and Teachers. The summary that you will compose will ensure that all participants have a common understanding of the child's personal and environmental challenges as well as the child's personal and environmental strengths. The COMPASS Challenges and Supports JSF will allow integration of data into an easy-to-read summary. This summary is used to guide the discussion during the COMPASS consultation. Before collating the data, be sure to obtain completed COMPASS Challenges and Supports Form for Caregivers and Teachers from both the caregiver and teacher.

Below are instructions on how to complete the COMPASS Challenges and Supports JSF.

1. Enter information on page 1 of the JSF. This includes student's name, date of birth, and date of consultation. Enter your name, the caregiver's name, special education teacher's name, and school name on the respective lines. Then summarize the child's personal information in the "Student's Likes, Strengths, Frustrations and Fears" section on the form (pp. 1–2 of the form). List items that both the caregiver and teacher find the student to like or be interested in. Also provide information on the child's strengths, frustrations, and fears.

2. Identify skills that are challenging for the student by using data that the teacher and caregiver provide on the "Adaptive Skills" section. Ratings of 3 and 4 on this form indicate difficult skills. Any time a caregiver or teacher rates a skill with a 3 or 4, place an "X" in the corresponding column.

3. The next section, "Problem Behaviors," utilizes the Problem Behavior Rating Scale. If a caregiver or teacher has marked any of these behaviors with a 3 or 4, place an "X" beside the behavior in the JSF.

4. In the "Social / Play Skills" section, place an "S"—indicating strength—in the corresponding box on the form for answers of 3 and 4. Place a "W"—indicating weakness—in the corresponding box on the form for answers of 1 and 2. Note: Be careful to place the "S" or "W" in appropriate box; placing an "S" or "W" in the incorrect box is easy to do and will result in an inaccurate depiction of the student's social abilities.

5. In the "Communication Skills" section, either write or type the examples provided by the caregiver and teacher. Another option is to photocopy the corresponding section of the COMPASS Challenges and Supports Form for Caregivers and Teachers and attach the copies to the JSF.

6. In the "Sensory Challenges" section, place a check mark in the corresponding box. Only items that are challenging are of interest in this section.

7. Summarize the student's "Sensory Supports." Place a check mark in the corresponding box that are supports or motivators for the student. Only items that are strengths or interests are of relevance in this section.

8. In the "Learning Skills" section, place an "S"—indicating strength—in the corresponding box on the form for answers of 3 and 4. Place a "W"—indicating weakness—in the corresponding box on the form for answers of 1 and 2. Note: Be careful to place the "S" or "W" in appropriate box; placing an "S" or "W" in the incorrect box is easy to do and will result in an inaccurate depiction of the student's social abilities.

9. The "Environmental Challenges" section can be used to make note of problems that are indicated on the forms or during the consultation.

10. The "Environmental Supports" section can be used to note any supports described in the forms or during consultation.

11. Finally, in the "Summary of Concerns" list the three concerns for each area as indicated by the caregiver and the teacher.

Appendix D   COMPASS Challenges and Supports Joint Summary Form

Child's/Student's Name: _____ Date of Birth: _____

Given by:

_____   _____
Consultant   Special Ed. Teacher

_____   _____
Caregiver   School

                                                              Date of Consultation:_____

1. Student's Likes, Strengths, Frustrations and Fears

Likes/Preferences/Interests:

Teacher: Caregiver:

Strengths or Abilities:

Teacher: Caregiver:

<u>Frustrations:</u>

Teacher: Caregiver:

<u>Fears:</u>

Teacher: Caregiver:

2. Personal Management/Adaptive Skills

These skills were marked as very difficult.

Self-management	Caregiver	Teacher
Performing basic self-care independently (such as toileting, dressing, eating, using utensils)		
Entertaining self in free time		
Changing activities—transitioning		
Sleeping		
Responding to Others	Caregiver	Teacher
Following 1 or 2 step direction		
Accepting "no"		
Answering questions		
Accepting help		
Accepting correction		
Being quiet when required		
Understanding Group Behaviors	Caregiver	Teacher
Coming when called to group		
Staying within certain places—lines, circles, chairs, desks		
Participating with the group		
Talking one at a time		
Picking up, cleaning up, straightening up, putting away		
Understanding Community Expectations	Caregiver	Teacher
Understanding who is a stranger		
Going to places in the community (place of worship, stores, restaurants, malls, homes)		
Understanding safety (such as streets, seat belts)		
Managing transportation (Cars/buses)		

3. Problem Behaviors*

These behaviors were marked as problematic	Teacher	Caregiver
1.	Acting impulsively, without thinking		
2.	Hitting or hurting others		
3.	Damaging or breaking things that belong to others		
4.	Screaming or yelling		
5.	Having sudden mood changes		
6.	Having temper tantrums		
7.	Having a low frustration tolerance; becoming easily angered or upset		
8.	Crying easily		
9.	Being overly quiet, shy, or withdrawn		
10.	Acting sulky or sad		
11.	Being underactive or lacking in energy		
12.	Engaging in behaviors that may be distasteful to others, such as nose-picking or spitting		
13.	Touching him/herself inappropriately		
14.	Engaging in compulsive behaviors; repeating certain acts over and over		
15.	Hitting or hurting him/herself		
16.	Becoming overly upset when others touch or move his/her belongings		
17.	Laughing/giggling at inappropriate times		
18	Ignoring or walking away from others during interactions or play		
19.	Touching others inappropriately		
20.	Engaging in unusual mannerisms such as hand-flapping or spinning		
21.	Having to play or do things in the same exact way each time		
22	Having difficulty calming him/herself down when upset or excited		
23.	Other: _____		

*Items are based on the Triad Social Skills Assessment

4. Social and Play Skills

How well does the child/student

Social Awareness	With adults		With children	
	Teacher	Caregiver	Teacher	Caregiver
1. Look toward a person who is talking to him/her				
2. Accept others being close to him/her				
3. Watch people for extended periods of time				
4. Respond to another person's approach by smiling or vocalizing				
5. Initiate interactions for social reasons				
Joint Attention Skills				
6. Look at something another person points to				
7. Show something to a person and look for person's reaction				
8. Point at an object or event to direct another person's attention to share enjoyment				
9. Share smile by looking back and forth between object and person				
Imitation				
10. Imitate sounds another person makes				
11. Imitate what another person does with an object (e.g., person makes toy airplane fly, child repeats action)				
12. Imitate body movements of others (such as clap when others clap, play Simon Says)				
13. Imitate and expand upon other's actions with toys (e.g., peer beats drum, child beats drum and also starts to march)				
Play				
14. Take turns within familiar routines (e.g., rolls a ballback and forth)				
15. Share toys				
16. Play interactively around a common theme				
17. Repair breakdowns during interactions (such as the child repeats or changes own behavior when other person seems confused or ignores)				
18. Pretends to do something or be something (such as that a plate is a hat by putting it on, to be a policeman, to have a tea party, that a doll is a teacher)				

5. Communication Skills

The following are descriptions of words or actions your child/student uses to communicate:

Making Requests	Teacher	Caregiver
1. Food		
2. Objects		
3. An activity		
4. To use the toilet		
5. Attention		
6. Help		
7. To play		
8. Information		
9. A choice		
Expressing Refusals	Teacher	Caregiver
1. "Go away"		
2. "No, I won't do it" or "I don't want it"		
3. "I want to be finished" or "I want to stop doing this"		
Expressing Thoughts	Teacher	Caregiver
1. Greeting to others		
2. Comments about people/ environment		
3. Confusion or "I don't know"		
4. Comments about errors or things wrong		
5. Asks about past or future events		
6. Agreement		

(continued)

(continued)

Expressing Feelings	Teacher	Caregiver
1. Angry/mad/frustrated		
2. Pain/illness/hurt		
3. Happy/excited		
4. Hurt feelings/upset		
5. Afraid		
6. Sad		

6. Sensory Challenges

These items were identified as being applicable to your child/student:

Sound/Auditory	Teacher	Caregiver
Has been diagnosed with hearing problem at some time	☐	☐
Reacts to unexpected sounds	☐	☐
Fears some noises	☐	☐
Distracted by certain sounds	☐	☐
Confused about direction of sounds	☐	☐
Makes self-induced noises	☐	☐
Fails to listen or pay attention to what is said to him/her	☐	☐
Talks a great deal	☐	☐
Own talking interferes with listening	☐	☐
Overly sensitive to some sounds	☐	☐
Seeks out certain noises or sounds	☐	☐
Other:_____	☐	☐
Taste	Teacher	Caregiver
Has an eating problem	☐	☐
Dislikes certain foods and textures	☐	☐
Will only eat a small variety of foods	☐	☐
Tastes/eats nonedibles	☐	☐
Explores environment by tasting	☐	☐
Puts most things in his/her mouth	☐	☐
Constant chewing on something	☐	☐
Other:_____	☐	☐
Sight/Vision	Teacher	Caregiver
Has trouble discriminating shapes, colors	☐	☐
Is sensitive to light—squints, wants to wear hats or sunglasses	☐	☐
Has trouble following with eyes	☐	☐
Does not make much eye contact	☐	☐
Is distracted by some or too much visual stimuli	☐	☐
Becomes excited when confronted with a variety of visual stimuli	☐	☐
Dislikes having eyes covered	☐	☐
Excited by vistas and open spaces	☐	☐
Hesitates going up or down stairs, curbs, or climbing equipment	☐	☐
Upset by things looking different (spills, spots)	☐	☐
Makes decisions about food, clothing, objects by sight	☐	☐
Closely examines objects or hands	☐	☐
Wants environment in certain order	☐	☐
Other:_____	☐	☐

(continued)

(continued)

Touch/Tactile	Teacher	Caregiver
Has to know someone is going to touch ahead of time	☐	☐
Dislikes being held or cuddled	☐	☐
Seems irritated when touched or bumped by peers	☐	☐
Explores environment by touching objects	☐	☐
Dislikes the feel of certain clothing	☐	☐
Refuses to touch certain things	☐	☐
Over or under dresses for the temperature or is unaware of temperature	☐	☐
Does not like showers or rain on self	☐	☐
Mouths objects or clothing	☐	☐
Refuses to walk on certain surfaces	☐	☐
Dislikes having hair, face, or mouth touched	☐	☐
Upset by sticky, gooey hands	☐	☐
Touches items with feet before hands	☐	☐
Does not like to hold hands	☐	☐
Pinches, bites, or hurts himself	☐	☐
Other:_____	☐	☐

Smell/Olfactory	Teacher	Caregiver
Sensitive to smells	☐	☐
Smells objects, food, people, toys more than usual	☐	☐
Explores environment by smelling	☐	☐
Reacts defensively to some smells	☐	☐
Ignores strong odors	☐	☐
Seeks out certain odors	☐	☐
Other:_____	☐	☐

Movement/Vestibular	Teacher	Caregiver
Seems fearful in space (teeter-totter, climbing)	☐	☐
Arches back when held or moved	☐	☐
Spins or whirls self around	☐	☐
Moves parts of body a great deal	☐	☐
Walks on toes	☐	☐
Appears clumsy, bumping into things and falling down	☐	☐
Avoids balance activities	☐	☐
Does not like to be around people in motion	☐	☐
Bumps into things and/or people	☐	☐
Other:_____	☐	☐

Visual/Perceptual Motor	Teacher	Caregiver
Has trouble with paper/pencil activities	☐	☐
Has difficulty with time perception	☐	☐
Has difficulty with body in space—moving appropriately	☐	☐
Has problems with use of some tools	☐	☐
Has problems organizing materials and moving them appropriately	☐	☐
Is distracted by doors and cupboards being open, holes, or motion	☐	☐
Other:_____	☐	☐

7. Sensory Supports

These items were identified as being applicable to your child/student:

Sound/Auditory	Teacher	Caregiver
Likes music	☐	☐
Likes to sing and dance	☐	☐
Taste		
Has definite eating preferences	☐	☐
Other:_____	☐	☐
Sight/Vision	Teacher	Caregiver
Enjoys watching moving things/bright objects	☐	☐
Enjoys patterns or shiny surfaces	☐	☐
Likes TV, videos, video games	☐	☐
Likes the computer	☐	☐
Other:_____	☐	☐
Touch/Tactile	Teacher	Caregiver
Likes to be touched	☐	☐
Likes hugs and cuddling when he/she initiates it	☐	☐
Likes to play in water	☐	☐
Likes baths or swimming pools	☐	☐
Seeks out mud, sand, clay to touch	☐	☐
Prefers deep touching rather than soft	☐	☐
Prefers certain textures of clothing	☐	☐
Likes being rolled or sandwiched between blankets/cushions	☐	☐
Likes rough and tumble play	☐	☐
Other:_____	☐	☐
Movement/Vestibular	Teacher	Caregiver
Enjoys rocking, swinging, spinning	☐	☐
Likes being tossed in the air	☐	☐
Likes to run	☐	☐
Likes and needs to move	☐	☐
Likes to climb; seldom falls	☐	☐
Other:_____	☐	☐
Visual/Perceptual Motor	Teacher	Caregiver
Relies on knowing location of furniture, stationary objects	☐	☐
Likes to draw and reproduce figures	☐	☐
Other:_____	☐	☐

8. Learning Skills

Learning/Work Skill	Caregiver	Teacher
1.	Child clearly understands the end goal of an activity, recognizes what he/she must do to be finished, and persists on the task to completion		
2.	Child realizes when he/she is running into difficulty and has some way of letting the adult know he/she needs help		
3.	Once an activity is under way, the adult can walk away from the child and he/she will keep working until finished, maintaining at least fairly good attention to what he/she is doing		
4.	Child finishes work and remembers on his/her own to let the adult know (e.g., by bringing work to adult, calling adult, raising his/her hand)		
5.	Child looks forward to earning a reward, knows it's next, work toward it, may ask for it or go get it on his/her own when work is finished		
6.	Child is able to wait briefly for a direction (anticipates that he/she is about to be asked to do something), is able to wait briefly for his/her turn with a toy (anticipating that it's about to return him/her), and / or wait for something to happen		
7.	Child may be distracted by outside sights and sounds or inner distractions (evident perhaps in singing to him/herself, gazing off, lining up materials) but is able to refocus attention to work on his/her own after a short time and without a prompt or reminder from the adult		
8.	Child shows interest in and curiosity about materials, handles them without prompting or nudging from the adult to get started. When one activity is finished he/she will look for another		
9.	Child can organize his/her responses to perform tasks when multiple materials are in front of him/her (e.g., a stack of cards for sorting)		
10.	Child recognizes when one strategy is not working and tries another way		
11.	Child recognizes his/her own mistakes and goes back and corrects them (e.g., takes little peg out of big hole to make room for correct peg)		

9. Environmental Challenges

Describe challenges noted in the Forms or reported during the consultation:

☐ Behavioral/Knowledge/Attitude of Other People Variables (such as inability to communicate clearly to the student, teach skills necessary for the activity, establish positive work or play routines).

☐ Procedural/Organizational (such as noisy environments, lack of visual supports, lack of effective transition routines).

☐ Temporal (such as lack or ineffective use of visual supports to understand passage of time or when activity is finished).

☐ Spatial (such as lack of personal space or clear boundaries).

10. Environmental Supports

Describe supports noted in the Forms or reported during the consultation:

☐ Behavioral/Knowledge/Attitude of Other People Variables (such as is able to communicate clearly to the student, teach skills necessary for the activity, establish positive work or play routines).

☐ Procedural/Organizational (such as uncluttered environments, visual supports for understanding work routines, positive transition routines).

☐ Temporal (such as visual supports to understand passage of time or when activity is finished).

□ Spatial (such as personal space to work and calm down, clear boundaries).

11. Summary of Concerns

Social and Play Skills

Teacher	Caregiver
1.	1.
2.	2.

Communication Skills

Teacher	Caregiver
1.	1.
2.	2.

Learning Skills

Teacher	Caregiver
1.	1.
2.	2.

Adaptive Skills

Teacher	Caregiver
1.	1.
2.	2.

Chapter 7
COMPASS Consultation Action Plan: Step B

Overview: Chapter 7 covers Step B of the COMPASS consultation process and provides forms and handouts used to conduct the consultation.

In this chapter, we:

1. Describe Part B of the COMPASS Consultation.
2. Prepare you to facilitate discussion of the parent's and teacher's concerns and generate consensus regarding prioritized skills.
3. Prepare you to write a measurable objective and a corresponding teaching plan.

The primary activity in this chapter sets the stage for developing the educational foundation for the student and is the second step described in the COMPASS Consultation Action Plan for Students with Autism (see Table 7.1). As you learned in Chap. 6, Step A helps the consultant prepare for the collaborative consultation. Chapter 7 provides a description of Step B, which is the beginning of the consultation process. The activities in Step B are designed to give all participants a common understanding of the student's current personal and environmental challenges and the personal and environmental supports necessary for success. It is encouraged that administrators and personnel who interact with the child be invited to the consultation. Although they may not have completed COMPASS forms, they will be able to provide valuable input and receive a wealth of information.

Step B: Activities During a COMPASS Consultation

Following the activities described in Step A in Chap. 6, activities in Step B focus on team building and discussion. The aim of Step B is for all participants to develop a shared understanding of the challenges (risk factors) to learning and the supports (protective factors) necessary for success for the particular student.

L.A. Ruble et al., *Collaborative Model for Promoting Competence and Success for Students with ASD*, DOI 10.1007/978-1-4614-2332-4_7, © Springer Science+Business Media, LLC 2012

Table 7.1 Step B of the COMPASS Consultation Action Plan for students with autism

1. Discuss COMPASS Consultation Training Packet
2. Discuss COMPASS Consultation Joint Summary
3. Identify and come to consensus on three prioritized objectives and write measurable objectives
4. Write measurable IEP objectives for the consensus areas
5. Develop COMPASS teaching plans for each measurable objective

In this chapter, we provide you with detailed instructions on how to conduct a COMPASS consultation. We have also included an *Abridged Protocol for Step B of the COMPASS Consultation Action Plan* in the forms section of this chapter. We recommend you print out this abridged version and take it with you to the consultation. This will help you keep focused and will help prompt you on the next steps.

The actions required in Step B are explained below.

Discuss COMPASS Consultation Training Packet

The COMPASS Consultation Training Packet provides the forms and illustrations of the concepts that you will use to generate a shared focus between the caregiver and teacher. Before you distribute the packet, you will first give a brief introduction of the goals and techniques of the consultation and will have participants sign in (see Section "Introduction and Sign In").

Introduction and Sign In

At the beginning of the consultation, introductions are provided and the role of the consultant is discussed (see Sample Script 1). We have provided sample scripts that can be used. When conducting the consultation, it is important that consultants apply their own style of interaction and use their own words. An important attribute of an effective consultant is authenticity.

Sample Script 1
Overview of COMPASS (show the COMPASS Model Form): "You know (student's name) better than I do. By working collaboratively using all of our knowledge and expertise, we can enhance (name's) response to his/her educational program. You have already provided us with a wealth of information about (student's name), which we will use today as we all plan together. I am here as a facilitator. I will be using the COMPASS Model to better understand (student's name) and develop a personalized program based on current best practices and your priorities for (student's name)" (Have participants sign COMPASS Sign In sheet).

Explanation of COMPASS

After the introduction, the consultant provides a copy of the set of materials labeled as the *COMPASS Consultation Training Packet* provided in the forms section at the end of the chapter. The training packet has handouts that are referred to during the consultation. First, an explanation of the model (see Sample Script 2) is provided.

Sample Script 2

Overview of COMPASS (show the COMPASS Model Form): "Our goal is to enhance (child's name) competence by considering how to balance personal and environmental challenges with personal and environmental supports. The challenges are the risk factors that may keep a student from learning. These include those within the child (personal factors) and those that the environment creates for the student (environmental factors). Supports are protective factors. They include personal strengths and interests and environmental supports such as teaching strategies and various accommodations or modifications. In order for a student to be successful there must be enough on the support side to balance what is on the risk side."

The consultant also refers to an *illustration of the COMPASS Model* (provided in the COMPASS Consultation Training Packet). The consultant should emphasize increasing the team's awareness of the relationship and the tentative balance between challenges and supports throughout the consultation. For example, the consultant reminds the team that the task of learning creates major stresses and anxieties for the child when the personal challenges combined with the environmental challenges are out of balance. The person with ASD is competent when the supports counterbalance the challenges. The role of the team, then, is to understand the process of how to identify, develop, implement, and monitor supports. As with all students, the supports or individualized instructional strategies need to be adjusted over time as the student develops and as environments change. To accomplish this goal successfully, the whole student has to be understood by all who are responsible for teaching the child and the consultant has to be able to help the parent and teacher understand the links between observable behavior, underlying symptoms of autism, and skills to teach.

Explanation of Purpose/Outcomes of COMPASS Consultation

After the basic information on the rationale of the approach for planning is explained and questions are answered, the consultant clarifies the purpose and expected outcomes of the consultation. The consultant then hands out the *Purpose/Outcomes of the COMPASS Consultation* sheet (see Table 7.2) and answers questions from the participants. This table is reproduced at the end of the chapter in a format suitable to give to the parent/caregiver and teacher.

Table 7.2 Purpose/outcomes of the COMPASS consultation

Enhance parent–teacher collaboration in order to provide a holistic assessment of the student's current functioning, learning, and needs
Provide a process to reach consensus on recommendations for an individualized educational program including specific positive, individualized teaching strategies
Write three measurable objectives from prioritized goals and develop specific teaching strategies for these. If preferred, the team may select to write more than three goals
Enhance purposeful and active student engagement in learning

Also provided is an *illustration of an iceberg* (available at the end of this chapter). This handout is used to illustrate two components that are critical during COMPASS consultation. The first aspect is to remind participants that the behaviors of children with autism represent the surface or tip of the iceberg. This is what we "see." As we share the information provided by the people who know and teach the child, we will be better able to examine what is happening below the surface, from the child's perspective. The child's behavior is influenced by the child's understanding of social interactions, ability to relate to others, understanding of language, and ability to communicate with others. Because children often cannot tell us what they are thinking or feeling, we have to interpret their thoughts and feelings. Our interpretation is based on what we are able to observe. But we also must be able to translate what we observe and act as an interpreter for the child.

The second aspect is that when there is behavior that is interfering with the child's progress toward developmental skills, an educational approach is taken to address the problem behavior. In other words, the goal is to identify what skills and knowledge the child needs to acquire to replace the problem behavior. Problem behaviors are viewed as serving some function for the student. Our job is to try to take the perspective of the student and understand how he or she views the world.

Overview of Best Practices

Next, the consultant provides an overview of best practices and distributes the *Overview of Best Practices for Individualized Education Plans* (*IEP*) *for Young Students with ASD handout* (see Table 7.3; also reproduced at the end of this chapter). This overview of best practices for educational programs comes from recommendations from the National Research Council (2001) for programs of children with autism between the age of 3 and 8 years.

It is helpful to educate or remind the caregivers and teachers of the components that are necessary for a high quality educational program. Also, it sets the stage for the rationale for developing IEP objectives that are essential for students with autism. One aim of the COMPASS consultation is the development of IEP objectives that address at minimum a social skill, a communication, and a learning skill. Learning skills are the behaviors that will assist the student in becoming more independent.

Table 7.3 Overview of best practices for individualized education plans (IEP) for young students with ASD

The Individualized Education Plan (IEP) is the method used for prioritizing and planning educational objectives. The educational objectives should include the growth of:

Social skills to improve involvement in school, family, and community activities (e.g., parallel and interactive play with family members and peers)

Expressive verbal language, receptive language, and nonverbal communication skills

A symbolic communication system that is functional when required

Engagement and flexibility in tasks and play that are developmentally appropriate. This should also include awareness of the environment and the ability to respond to appropriate motivational systems

Fine and gross motor skills to be utilized when engaging in age-appropriate activities

Cognitive or thinking skills, which include academic skills, basic concepts, and symbolic play

Replacement of problem behavior with more conventional or appropriate behavior

Behaviors that are the foundation to success in a regular classroom (following instructions, completing a task) and independent organizational skills

Discuss the COMPASS Consultation Joint Summary

After these activities, the consultant provides the participants a copy of the COMPASS Consultation Joint Summary forms previously completed by the parents/caregivers and teachers and summarized using the *Joint Summary Template* (at the end of the chapter). The next step is the identification of the parents' and teachers' concerns and priorities, followed by agreement on at least three teaching objectives that address social skills, communication skills, and learning skills. Each skill is translated into a specific and measurable teaching objective. Chapter 5 discusses in more detail how to write IEP objectives that are of high quality. The last activity is the development of COMPASS teaching plans for each measurable objective. Each one of the four activities is described below and more detail is provided.

Specifically, the consultant will review summary information from the parent and teacher COMPASS forms and provide copies of the summary to all participants. This step is performed by sharing with the participants the information from teacher and parent forms, showing how this information fits in the model, asking if it looks accurate, and finding out if there is other information to add.

As the consultant, you are responsible for keeping the team focused and moving forward. Summarize information as it is shared and remind the participants of the link between what they are observing and how their observations relate to the COMPASS model. It is helpful to take notes throughout and keep in mind issues that the caregiver and teacher describe as salient. Also, keep in mind pivotal skills that might be important for selection as a targeted objective. Table 7.4 provides ideas on how the consultant can keep the team focused and moving forward during the consultation.

The review begins with a discussion of the *child's strengths and preferences* (see Fig. 7.1), followed by *fears and frustrations*. Be sure to obtain examples of behaviors and use this information to help the participants understand that the child may not

Table 7.4 Ideas on how to keep the team focused during the consultation

Clarify questions and concerns
  A. Ask open-ended questions
  B. Paraphrase what is said
  C. "Listen" for feelings
Keep the group moving and focused
  A. Attend to the time involved for each aspect of the consultation and monitor allotted time throughout consultation
  B. Allow enough time for information to be shared, but not so much time that all activities are not completed
  C. Gently redirect conversations that stray from the goal of the activity
Involve all participants
  A. Steer dominant participants to listen
  B. Ask open-ended questions and seek information from quiet participants
  C. Summarize concerns as a topic area closes
Value all participants' input
  A. Remain nonjudgmental
  B. Use attentive and open body posture
  C. Use gestures, nods, and facial expressions to communicate attending
  D. Use minimal encouragers
  E. Use a tone of voice that communicates interest
Question members effectively to draw ideas from group
  A. Ask questions that relate to the topic and are open ended
  B. Use Socratic questioning techniques
  C. Avoid giving answers and instead ask questions
  D. Avoid acting as "expert"
Be flexible enough to include unexpected information
  A. Adjust allotted time to address issues or concerns that arise
  B. Prioritize time to address unexpected information
  C. Validate concerns
Summarize as group moves along
  A. Summarize information before moving on to new topic or area of discussion
  B. Rephrase information in your own words

be able to express emotions directly and must rely on behavior to do so. Behaviors may be expressions of frustration that must be interpreted by others. The iceberg model is helpful in making the connection between observable behaviors and underlying skill deficits.

The next section covered is *adaptive skills*. It is important to obtain a sense of how much of a problem these issues are and for teachers to understand what the issues are outside the classroom. Often, this activity reminds teachers of the stress that parenting a child with autism may pose and the necessity of teaching adaptive skills that impact everyday living (Fig. 7.2).

M = Mom; T = Teacher; C = Consultant

C: You have marked that he likes to be touched.

M: He's super at hugging and cuddling.

C: He likes water, rough and tumble play, enjoys walking and swimming and jumping.

T: Well, I didn't mark walking, swimming or spinning like his mom did because I don't usually have him do those things. I mean he'll bounce, he'll jump…

C: Okay.

M: And I don't put those in the same context of, to me those of stimming behaviors or characteristics. I don't correlate him doing it in a stimming manner.

C: Right.

M: He's definitely a mobile kid.

C: And you listed computer games, reading, board games.

M: He constantly reads, he almost compulsively reads.

T: Yes. It's to the point that he will read anything that's around him. Anything that you have posted that is within his line of sight.

C: So that is a distracter for him?

M: Yes, and he will read like the teacher directions, like all the fine print…

T: Fine print kind of interests him because he thinks that it's some kind of secret something. He pays close attention to visual details.

M: He completely taught himself to read at age two. I mean we've always read to him but we never had to teach him anything with reading.

T: He's very photographic about it. He's not very phonetic about it so he's been stumbling with some words that you say to him that are not phonetic. Like he has that visual recall of the word.

M: And with that visual recall of the word it's very interesting because conversationally I can tell that he's pronouncing a word the way he's seeing it. He's a highly visual learner and poor auditory learner.

C: Mmm

M: My husband said "I kind of always thought of his reading as his stimming behavior." It is a self calming tool for him and now he always utilizes it.

T: He's reading every time he is on a self break. He will give himself a self break where he can go read.

C: Is his comprehension on par with his reading?

T: Not particularly. He can pronounce most anything. He can decode just about anything we put in front of him. He just doesn't have the maturity to comprehend middle school material.

C: Yes

T: When he is upset he comes in here and bounces on the ball and reads the Cheerio box while I am talking to him.

C: So he's choosing reading for a lot of reasons. It's therapeutic. It's used as a stim to calm down. It's a distracter. It is everywhere and he reads everything. He pulls into himself.

M: And in a way, I mean my husband and I both read a ton, too. And in a way I can relate to it very much. It is, you know, it's after a stressful day. You cannot think about it and I think that's exactly what he's using reading for.
Subject is changed:

C: So all your hard work of filling the forms out has paid off. What do you have to do to make sure he is engaged?

Fig. 7.1 Excerpt from consultation on examples of strengths and preferences that leads to further discussion of behavior

M = Mom; T = Teacher; C = Consultant

T: And you know he pitches a fit in the bathroom for you to pull up his pants. You have to coach him for him to do it. He can do it, but he wants you to do it. And if you don't do it he comes at you and says, "Want help" or "You do it" or something to get you to pull them up. When I say, "No" he makes warning noises.

C: So some of what we want him to do is be independent at doing the things he can do. We need something for this I think. It is a big part of kindergarten.

T: I don't know if it is a control thing or not. He's controlling you by telling you to pull up his pants.

C: Well, I think there is another part here too that you were talking about earlier. He can do things but wants you in the room.

T: and M: Right.

M: He is dependent upon the praise.

T: We need to get him to do it without the praise.

C: Without a lot of constant attention. Or figure out how he can reward himself and show us later at a different time. "Look what I did! I did it by myself!" He could learn to do that.

M: Yes, or give yourself a hand.

C: So, we can find an objective that would hit at these things... It is kind of like self-monitoring, doing things with self regulation. He might have a little checklist that is on his desk. He gives himself a check or happy face if he did the things on the list.

T: Good idea.

C: But there have to be teacher reliability checks to say, "You're right, I agree with you." And it might just be, "Look at what you did! We are going to show Mom!"

T: Mmm, because he does go home and show her things that he did during the day.

M: He has not done that until this year. Sometimes he tells me. Like when I say, "How was your day?" He might say, "The playground, Ms Joy kick!" You know he has it going on in his head.

T: You have to read between the lines to figure out that he did something.

M: At least he is trying to let you know, last year you got nothing out of him.

C: So, it's almost like in our three goals that there is group behaviors, this whole thing about self monitoring, and then peer interaction.

T: And how is that going to work? They are not taken directly from the IEP.

C: Two are directly from the IEP and one you will probably need to add.

T: OK, because that is how we need to monitor progress, correct?

C: Right.

Fig. 7.2 Excerpt from COMPASS consultation on coming to agreement on helping the child reach more independence while discussing behavior and relating to goals

Related to personal management are *problem behaviors*. During this review, obtain a sense of how interfering the behaviors are and make note of these behaviors. As information is shared on the child's social and communication skills, making a link between these problem behaviors and skill deficits using the iceberg model will help identify pivotal skills that can replace problem behaviors (Fig. 7.3).

The next session deals more directly with the *child's play and social skills*. Understanding how the child plays and interacts with objects provides important information that can be used to help participants interpret why the child may not be interacting or playing with other children appropriately. It also helps them understand where the child is starting before the next step of skill development can occur and that specific teaching plans will need to be implemented to obtain the next step.

M = Mom; T = Teacher; C = Consultant; Adm = Administrator

C: What is a tantrum? If I saw a tantrum on videotape what would it look like? What does he do first? The first sign?

T: Screaming, he does that "AHHH"

M: It's that scream.

T: Yes, Well sometimes it's that he stiffens up and stops. He just stops where he is and ofcourse he weighs 80lbs, so it's like...I can't get him to go.

M: The last we weighed at the doctor's office which wasn't that long ago, about a month, he was 56 lbs.

T: Which is big. (Laughs)

M: He's stocky.

T: He stiffens and stops and does that vocalizing, kind of like an EHHH. And then it's yelling out and if it's really bad it's the screaming, the pulling away, the jerking away and then there were a couple of times where there's just been tears, just the crying, and he's really loud.

C: So that's a tantrum that can also go into aggression?

Adm: Well, that's the wailing out loud on the floor...does it lead into that?

T: Yea. The aggression...I don't know. It's just kind of hard to put a finger on this. It's kind of like the jerking away and the pulling because I really haven't seen the aggression this year. That day he laid his hand on my cheek was the most aggressive thing he's done.

C: That's a good thing.

T: Last year he would lunge at me and try to bite me and I haven't seen that. Even though his frustration level has increased significantly, his aggression has decreased.

C: How many times at school on an average day would you say he has one of these episodes?

T: Full blown or just a portion of?

C: Any portion.

T: Oh, gosh... 10 to 15

M: Oh my gosh, I didn't know it was that bad.

T: Well, it's just whenever it's time to come in from a walk or it's time to come in from the playground and he's not ready to come in or if it's time to go back and do tasks, it's kind of like..

C: What does he do to protest since it isn't the full blown tantrum?

T: It's kind of jerking away, stopping and it's more vocalizations, EEH! But it's really loud. It's not necessarily screaming or yelling but it's a really loud vocalization.

Adm: Will he give in and do it?

T: Most of the time.

Adm: Like if you redirect him it stops the fit?

T: Most of the time. If you say, "No. This is not a choice. Line up," he'll do it. He'll go on and do it, but full blown....

C: Full blown, How many of those a day?

T: There's probably not an average of 1 a day.

C: And that's where he's on the ground?

T: Right, Yea.

C: And those are the ones that last for some time?

T: MMM. To me maybe two or three standout since school has started. Again where it was really hard to get him to calm down. He was just in tears and he was just so upset that it was hard to kind of get him to chill out a little bit.

C: Would you say a couple a week?

T: Full blown. No

C: Once a week?

T: Maybe at the most

Fig. 7.3 Excerpt from consultation—discussion of trying to understand behavior

M = Mom; T = Teacher; C = Consultant; Adm = Administrator

C: What about at home?

Adm: I know his grandma said he had one this weekend that lasted twenty minutes.

C: Does that sound like the full blown tantrum we have talked about and is that what you see at home?

M: MMMMM

C: Is there aggression at home?

M: Not a whole lot.

C: Do you get a lot of this protesting at home?

M: Yes, Oh, yes.

C: But not as much as a full blown tantrum?

T: But at home I think too, and I think mom would agree, is a lot less structured than at school.

M: Yes

T: He doesn't have a set bedtime. He doesn't sit down to eat supper at a set time necessarily. There's not nearly the structure he has here.

Adm: Same time we eat breakfast, same time we eat lunch.

C: When he is having a tantrum at home, not full blown, how many times do you say that happens like during an evening.

M: A lot. I mean anytime... but I don't make him..

C: So if you ask him or tell him to do anything it would be a tantrum?

M: Yes

C: And then what happens?

M: Going to bed has been really hard. Last week he didn't go to bed until 12 or 12:30 and I couldn't get him to lay down.

T: Which in turn affects him at school because he comes in and from the moment he hits the door it's, "Whoa, he's in a bad mood today."

C: So pretty much every night bedtime is a hard time?

M: Except the last two nights he has been in bed at 10:30.

T: But does he still get up during the middle of the night and wander around?

M: Sometimes. He does it regularly, but it's not everyday. It's like once every two weeks.

C: What about getting him up in the morning?

M: Oh, it's hard.

C: And dressing him...

M: I try to wake him up. I'm like Jimmy, let's get ready for school. Get up. Get up. He won't. I physically have to lift him up.

C: That's every day? Every morning?

M: Mmm.

C: And do you dress him?

M: Yes

C: OK. And is he protesting.

M: He's asleep.

C: OK so really at home it's hard to ask him to do anything.

M: Uh Huh.

C: So we are really talking a lot about motivation and trying to figure out how to get him to want to follow our directions.

Adm: For safety reasons too. You know...not to run out of the cafeteria and into the parking lot.

C: So let's identify things that make him mad or upset. These are the triggers to his behaviors. And we have talked about running off, jerking away, refusing to move, and tantrums.

T: He screams when we take him to the potty, when he has to come in, when he has to stop doing something he likes, when he has to sit...

C: OK, when you are requiring him to stop something to transition to something else, transition times...

T: It's more like a transition from a preferred activity to a non-preferred.

C: Right. It seems like he does the folder time without protest.

Fig. 7.3 (continued)

M = Mom; T = Teacher; C = Consultant; Adm = Administrator

T: Yes, because it's the one time where he's made to sit down and focus. We are going to make an exact schedule with pictures for him.

C: How many folders will he do now?

T: He will do five, but not without some fussing and trying to get out of it.

C: But can he do them?

T: Oh, yes. And that's what's so upsetting, I've seen his potential. He is just like a little sponge.

C: When is he trying to get away from you?

T: Well he is in a corner blocked in with someone sitting behind him straddling him in a chair so he can't go anywhere. All his choice is to sit there and yell. Sometimes he'll flop and try to slide down under the table. You have to straddle him and hold your feet up against the chair so he can't scoot it and wrap your legs around it. This is becoming a real disturbance to the other children.

C: Well, let's look at this. You are wanting to teach him and you are wanting his tantrums to decrease. What do you want to see increase? Compliance?

T: Yes, I want him to comply.

C: So what I am thinking of are the skills we want to teach him. So staying calm...

T: Appropriate communication... functional communication.

C: Well, what if he communicated "No" instead of screaming and yelling? He just said, "No."

T: Right. Yea. Which we still can't always... even if he says "No" he might still have to do it.

C: Right now it looks like he is turning away, screaming and tantrumming for all negations on this sheet, "I don't want to," "Go away," "No, I won't," "I don't want it," "I want to be finished." So, maybe that's what we want to do. Teach him a functional way to indicate "No." It doesn't mean giving in to him, it means we got his message and then in a minute he will do the activity.

T: He also may need more choice.

Adm: He could choose "Yes." He could choose from a card like "Want to be alone," "Going to a special place," "Going for a walk," etc.

C: OK, so I added on here, saying "No." But then we need to motivate him to complete something even though it is frustrating to him. And we will addmaking choices.

Fig. 7.3 (continued)

The questions that ask about the *social behaviors with adults and with children* are intended to help the participants "see" that the children interact with adults better than with children. The consultant explains that adults tend to structure social situations for the child and adapt more to the child than peers do. Because of this, specific teaching plans will need to consider peer interactions and peer training. See Fig. 7.4 for an excerpt of discussion on social and play skills from a consultation.

Analysis of *communication skills* occurs next. The consultant reviews the words and actions the child uses to make specific requests, to negate, to comment and to express feelings. During this review, the consultant can emphasize the extent to which the child relies on behaviors and actions to communicate the messages. Figure 7.5 provides the dialogue between the participants on gaining consensus on how to use a visual communication system. Discussion also needs to include pivotal communication skills to target in the educational plan. If the child has significant behaviors that interfere with learning and participation in home and school activities, analyze possible communicative intentions of the problem behavior. Again, refer to the iceberg model and question participants' theories about the causes of behavior. For example, if the child refuses to complete a requested activity, examine how it is that the child expresses no or refusal. If the child hits or scratches when given a request, this suggests a pivotal skill for the child to learn—how to indicate no appropriately (Fig. 7.5).

M = Mom; T = Teacher; C = Consultant; Sp Path = Speech Language Pathologist	
C:	So, when he's playing with other children, he's playing mostly alongside them?
T:	Yes.
M:	He will go get somebody on the playground to teeter totter with him because he knows that requires two.
C:	That's great. How does he do that?
T:	He'll just grab them.
C:	What if they don't want to?
T:	We tell them that Gary wants you to teeter totter. And they are like okay with that. Gary wants me to teeter totter. He doesn't want to do it for a long, long time. They'll just stop what they're doing and go do it. Gary gets off and everyone is happy.
C:	Well the other kids must like to do it too.
T:	Yes. They love him.
M:	He's very affectionate and easy-going for the most part.
C:	And some of the ways he plays with his cousin is to rough house?
M:	Yes, they are playing. They're wrestling and they're laughing. Sometimes we have to tell them, "No more."
C:	Yes, roll balls or something else. So now let's go for a minute to imitation, because that is an important pivotal skill that children need to have in order to learn.
T:	We clearly have Gary doing that by watching the other children and doing what they are doing so he can imitate body movements, sounds, what a kid does with an object.
C:	Many children with autism don't have these skills at his age. So he has this basic skill that is going to help all of his learning. Now let's look at interactions for a minute. You say that he interacts with both adults and peers but there are some problems keeping interactions going. Is he doing much cooperative play - going back and forth with children?
Sp Path:	I don't see much cooperative play.
C:	It's more parallel from what you describe.
T:	Yes, It's more parallel. He builds nice roads out of blocks and stuff but not really with anybody. Now, I've had him do it before. I say, "Let's build" and do it with him, and he will.
C:	So with help he will do it.
T:	Yes, I'll say, "Come on guys, let's build," and so he'll come and do that.
M:	He's getting better, but when he first started he would stick to himself a lot.
T:	Yes, and he still does.
C:	And what about his turn-taking in general?
T:	We're working on it.
M:	If the baby picks up anything of his or even touches it he's like, "No baby," and he gets mad and the baby is just getting big enough to be able to do that.
C:	And well, it may have to be that some things are Gary's, and some are baby's, and some are to be shared.
M:	He imitates what he sees on TV. I caught him doing that dance the other day. He loves play station too.
C:	So he has some very good social skills to build on. Maybe taking turns with peers might be something to work on.

Fig. 7.4 Excerpt on discussion of social/play skills from COMPASS consultation

The next two sections cover *sensory challenges and sensory supports*. Because young children with autism have limited ways to express themselves, it may be difficult to understand what types of environmental stimuli may bother them. What bothers one child may not bother another child with autism. Thus, sensory challenges are environmental risk factors personalized to each child. They need to be

M = Mom; T = Teacher; C = Consultant

M: We have tons of cards at home. He's got the first set and the second set. We go through them.

C: Well maybe there are some that he uses at home that he doesn't use at school.

M: Well sure.

C: I wonder if we can't combine and use the cards in some way. We really want him to begin to communicate with other children. So like "Will you chase me?" - knowing the chase card and taking it to another child so he can play chase since this a preferred activity.

T: Yes, we can think of ways for him to communicate with other kids with the cards.

M: OK, say like for instance, he was pulling at the little girl for her to play. Instead of pulling at the little girl, say "Joey, what do you want the little girl to do?" He could choose from two cards, and you could say, "Do you want to go on the playground with her or play ball with her?"

T: So he will show a card?

M: You know he will show swing, he'd be there all the time. He uses a trampoline a lot too.

C: Yes, I think it can be the same format that he's got here, but needs to use it with peers because that seems to be a challenge for him.

M: I am struggling with that.

C: It will take training of his peers too. I think that he is with a wonderful class of children.

T: I agree. I mean if he went up and said, "I want a swing" and if he went to the swings and they were full and the kids saw Jerry head to the swing, they will get off and let him have it.

M: Oh, that's not fair.

T: But that's okay.

C: But that would be neat for him to go up to someone and communicate, "I want a swing."

M: That would make them feel really good too, "Oh, wow! OK, Jerry just talked to me!"

T: Oh, of course!

C: And they have been able to help, and that's the way Jerry talks.

T: And we have discussed it with them.

C: And I think too that when you are watching you can figure out what he needs to say back. Right now he does not have a way to say something back.

T: Right

C: The kids may give you some more ideas about what pictures to put on there.

T: They do. They talk to him. They love to look through the pictures and are so intrigued. They just think it is really neat.

C: So, that's perfect. We've got children who are going to be fantastic at doing this. So how do we write this into an objective.

T: If you don't ask the question the right way, he can't answer it.

C: You already have this on his IEP. Jerry will initiate social interaction. So let's say, Jerry will initiate communication with peers. Right? That is what we're wanting him to do?

T: Uh huh.

M: Yes.

C: Jerry will initiate communication with peers using his communication system, 4 of 5times a day?

T: You have to have a number attached to it, so how many times? It has to be measureable. So I would look at it as the person who is outdoors with him, would tell me how many times this week he used his card to request out on the playground.

C: So he has someone with him on the playground all the time?

T: Yes. Then we've got to have him carry it with him where he goes.

C: And we want him to do this independently, in other words, without being cued. But do we have to put one with adult cues and then the next one with peer cues? Do you need to tier...

M: Oh, I see exactly what you're saying.

T: Like with the hierarchy.

C: Yes.

Fig. 7.5 Excerpt on discussion of gaining consensus on how to use a visual communication system that leads to discussion of goal and teaching strategies

M = Mom; T = Teacher; C = Consultant

T: I don't know on the IEP…

C: Okay, so, I'll tell you what, let's do it that way. We'll start with the adult cue, because he's probably going to need to be cued within the teaching strategy.

T: Yes.

C: Because he's going to go pull the little girl, since he knows that is what works. So why use something else when this works? The little girl and the other kids in the class are going to have to know to cue him and not just let him have the swing.

T: Right

C: So, let's say with verbal or physical cues, so that means that he gets the cues from the kids or adult cues. The next one would be written independently at which point you're probably going to have to retrain the children to know to wait and not cue him.

T: Yeah, that's kind of like what we do naturally.

C: Like with the cue, "Tell me what you want Jerry?" Other kids will be able to do that. Does that sound right? And we will write all this out in detail.

T: We put both of them together?

C: Well I have… Jerry will initiate interaction with peers using his communication system four or five times daily in two different situations (i.e. playground, certain center, snack time) with visual cues and no more than two adult verbal cues - then with peer cues for the next one. And then the next one is going to be written independently with visual cues only. Once he gets to 4 of 5 times on the first one, we move to the next one. What are the personal challenges for him to be able to do this, to reach this? What do we know that will make this hard for him?

T: I've begun to back off a little and let him be a little bit more independent on the playground and not have to have that adult right with him. And that may be one reason why we're seeing him doing a little more initiating because that adult is backing off and not running or climbing and being the playmate with him. He needs to go out and search for other people himself.

M: Now one thing, there's not playmates that live close to us or anything.

T: I know, in his class, that there would be a great child that would …

C: That's an environmental challenge. Not many peers at home.

M: Uh, huh.

C: Peers for him to interact with. He's got a whole lot of other supports but not peers. What other kind of challenges, personal challenges?

T: Well, he's got habits, he's got to learn to replace behaviors.

C: Exactly. When he goes to pull and it doesn't work then, we need something for the frustration.

M: There will be withdrawals probably.

C: Right.

M: With frustration.

C: So having the prompt will help, and it would be great if it could come from the peer or whomever is right there.

T: And I have been using it some. "Jerry that's fine. Jerry don't pull me. Use your words." I got that from his speech teacher.

C: What do you say to him, "Use your words?"

M: I say, "Show me what you want." "Yeah, that's fine." "Use your words." "Show me, where's your book?" And his book stays on the kitchen table at home all the time. That's where it stays because it is at eye level. That's the spot he chose to put it. And he will go get it and bring it to me and show me when he is in other parts of the house.

C: Great, great

M: But he's pretty independent at home. He just goes to the refrigerator and gets his own drink…

C: And that's one of the challenges we find with children with autism. It is much harder to communicate through somebody than to go and get it myself or do it myself.

M: Uh, huh.

Fig. 7.5 (continued)

considered and addressed when developing the teaching plan so that learning is not hindered.

Sensory supports like sensory challenges are also individualized for each child. Because many young children are at the sensory and motor level of development, activities and objects that have a sensory component can be used for increasing motivation to complete tasks. Building sensory supports into the child's program can also help with maintaining the child's attention to tasks. See Fig. 7.6 excerpt on a discussion of sensory challenges and supports.

M = Mom; T = Teacher; C = Consultant; Sp Path = Speech and Language Pathologist; Adm = Administrator	
C:	Let's talk about her sensory needs. You have a number of items marked in the auditory area. She makes self-induced sounds. She has problems paying attention. She's sensitive to some sounds and she seeks out some sounds. What noises is she more sensitive to and which does she seek out?
T:	At school she's sensitive to crying and screeches, like in the lunchroom - like when they are putting up the tables before we are done eating. Anything that is out of the ordinary especially in a big room that echoes. Sounds she seeks out are rhythm, pops, bubbles popping, and music. We do rhythm sticks and she really likes that. So anything that is constant and steady, she seeks that out. I notice a lot of songs that she likes. They all have that same beat. Did you notice that?
M:	No, I didn't notice that. I just know that she likes them.
T:	Like, Pop-pop-pop! That one..the beat!
C:	With sight or vision she likes moving things and is excited by open spaces. She likes TV, she likes the computer. Is she distracted by too much visual stimuli and do you see patterns at school?
T:	No.
C:	She doesn't make much eye contact, which both of you said and she has trouble following with her eyes. She does not track well?
M:	Not normally, no.
C:	She explores with her hands and fingers. Touches things a lot. She likes water, mouthing things. She's not too aware if she is hurt, you have marked.
M:	If something hurts, she is getting to where she will show me. She can't really tell me that her stomach hurts, but if she hurts her foot, she comes to me and sticks her foot in my face.
C:	Yes, Anything else with tactile? She seems irritated when bumped by peers.
M:	She doesn't like it when other kids touch her, that I have noticed. Does she do that at school?
T:	Well, we don't touch her.
M:	Well, I saw a kid when I was here who was touching her. She was kind of like pushing her buttons. She turned around and looked at her like she was kind of scared, like she didn't understand. She just looks at them funny when they touch her.
C:	But she likes hugs and cuddling. Does she initiate that?
M:	Yes.
C:	You have a lot of things around taste. Where she dislikes certain textures and foods. What textures does she like and what does she dislike?
M:	Well, she eats chicken and dumplings and they are kind of slimy. And then she likes Cheetos that are real hard and kind of crunch. So I don't know. She loves macaroni and cheese - that is squishy.

Fig. 7.6 Excerpt on discussion of reviewing the sensory checklist and considering what sensory preferences might be used as supports. There is some frustration about the sensory problems

M = Mom; T = Teacher; C = Consultant; Sp Path = Speech and Language Pathologist; Adm = Administrator

C: What does she really not like?
M: She never really... she doesn't try anything new.
T: She tried that Jello once.
M: I think she just plays with it. We do that in restaurants. I just get her a big plate of Jello, and she plays with it until I am done eating. I think she thinks it is a toy.
C: That's a good strategy.
M: She eats mostly breads and cheese. Stuff like that.
Sp Path: No fruits, right?
T: I thought she eats grapes?
M: Does she?
T: She tried a few at school. I cut them up real small and she licked them first.
M: She used to eat apples with cinnamon and sugar on them but not now.
C: And the other issue is putting things in her mouth. She mouths a lot of things?
M: Everything
Sp Path: But don't you think that is much improved?
M: Oh, definitely.
Adm: Last year it was a constant. Somebody constantly had to be with her to make sure that she wasn't putting things in her mouth. Now we don't have to watch that closely.
T: Now it's more exploratory. She'll touch it with her tongue but not really put it in her mouth.
M: Sometimes she tries to rub her tongue on someone's head.
T: Especially a little guy in the class with a buzz cut and she loves to touch it and lick it. It's a comforting thing and he lets her rub all she wants to. Last year it was such a worry since she would put the smallest anything in her mouth.
M: She does taste the shaving cream, but spits it out.
C: So she is not ingesting any of it. Let's look at movement. She seems fearful on the teeter totter and climbing.
T: On our climbing gym outside there are little tiny holes in it and the perception seems to be a little off, and she is fearful of that. Someone has to be right there with her. But she is better than last year.
C: And she spins herself. She enjoys rocking, walking on her toes.
T: I haven't noticed much toe walking.
M: She doesn't do it all the time, but sometimes she does. Not constant.
C: What of these sensory items does she like to do? Which are preferences for her that can be used for supports and reinforcement? They are helpful for her.
Sp Path: Swinging.
M: We have a toddler swing at home and she loves it.
T: She sorts the legos and finds the yellow ones.
M: She likes toys that feel really weird.
T: She likes the rocking chair in our room too, comfort. It's a thing she does on her own. She also likes to run her fingers over strings that are hanging and watch them move.
M: She likes toys from her video.
T: She likes Dora
C: So she likes videos?
M: We rotate them. She has so many. She doesn't have to watch the same one. She doesn't seem to care which she watches.
C: Then she likes the figures that she has seen in the video?
M: I go in there and sing and point with them. It's what we do.
Sp Path: It is so hard to find motivators for her.

Fig. 7.6 (continued)

The final domain of discussion is *learning skills*. Learning skills are the underlying adaptive classroom skills that help children become more independent and effective problem solvers. These are core skill areas impaired like social and communication skills. It is important to discuss with the participants how weaknesses in learning skills affect all areas of learning and independence. Also, if the child has a teaching assistant, helping participants understand that the teaching assistants can become environmental risks when they take over and perform these skills for the child. As this information is shared, the consultant should keep cognizant of which learning skills are emerging and what might be targeted in the educational plan (Fig. 7.7).

M = Mom; T = Teacher; C = Consultant

M: She likes to be unnoticed.

C: She's got to be independent when she wants to do it without anybody looking or interfering with her, right?

T: That's just the thing with her. We know she can do these things but she won't when asked to.

C: She may want to know that she can do it right.

T: Yes.

C: She's not going to get started unless she knows exactly…

M: Laughs…Maybe

C: So you want her to start an activity independently.

T: An activity not of her choosing when requested.

C: And is the request verbal, gestural, visual?

T: She does it now, hand-over-hand.

C: Now she holds her ears and whines when she may want something so the adult has to do all the interpreting. The challenge is that she is a very low initiator. She has to rely on routines and she keeps doing things the same way she is used to doing them.

M: But her brother can get her to imitate him and do things with him.

C: So a peer she trusts and knows is a good model for her. I think that another challenge is that she doesn't have a lot of things that she wants.

T: She is just content to be passive. She's pretty busy in her head.

C: Well, she kind of entertains herself in her head.

M: And she is very cute, and it is easy for her to get adults to do things for her.

C: Is that an environmental challenge or an adult problem? It's a support that she is cute, but it may get in the way of learning.

T: And when she whines, people want to give in to her.

M: But don't (laughs).

C: She needs a model and demonstration, and she needs routine that she can depend on.

T: So in our small group she can see the materials, see how to do the activity from me and a peer, and we do this every day, not always the same thing, but something similar. I will make sure she knows what to do before directing her to do it.

M: She spends a lot of time at home just watching her brother and sister.

Fig. 7.7 Excerpt of discussion of learning skills during a COMPASS consultation

Identify and Come to a Consensus on the Top Three Concerns

Review the summary concerns form that was provided to the participants. Remind the parent and teacher that these concerns become the priority skills for the child to learn. Emphasize that a social skill, a communication skill, and a learning skill are to be targeted for the educational plan because these skills set the foundation for higher level skills. If the child has problem behaviors, help the participants understand the links between the observable (problem) behavior and the underlying impairments in autism that are influencing the behavior. Case study 1 provides a detailed example of how this was done for one child, Anthony.

As the teacher and caregiver concerns are shared with the team, it is helpful for the consultant to write the primary concerns on a whiteboard or paper that the team can view together. The consultant explains and shows the areas of concern that overlap as well as the areas that are distinct. It is likely that most of the concerns will be expressed by both the caregiver and teacher. Skills that may not overlap may be domains of learning that are a relative priority at school (academic skills) or at home (adaptive skills). Acknowledge the importance of these skills but also explain that the focus is to gain consensus on the skills that relate to the domains of social, communication, and learning skills. If there are differences in perceptions of what the priority should be, remind the team of the notion of pivotal skills that when learned, have widespread effects on other areas of development. Figure 7.8 is an excerpt of a discussion on coming to consensus for a social skill goal during a COMPASS consultation combined with writing the goal.

M = Mom; T = Teacher; C = Consultant; Sp Path = Speech and Language Pathologist	
C:	These were some of the concerns you listed and we are going to come to some consensus on the main ones we are going to work on. Some of her main social challenges are tolerating others, interacting / communicating with peers, playing, and moving beyond parallel play. So out of those what would you target to be the main one you feel we need to work on with social skills as we break it down into measurable goals?
T:	I think actual interactions with and communicating with peers.
M:	See all of this plays into that as far as I see it.
T:	'Cause now at this point tolerating others, playing in a circle she is doing great. So a lot of it is learned behavior once she becomes comfortable.
C:	So do you see some kind of reciprocal interaction with peers being targeted as a goal?
T:	Yes.
M:	That would be wonderful!
T:	You can just say initiating, like a verbal 'Come do this with me.' Some kind of initiating play - but that's just the first step I guess.
C:	We can also look at putting something in as a communication skill. If she says, 'Come play with me,' she's got to be able to do something with play.
T:	Right, right.

Fig. 7.8 Excerpt on discussion of coming to consensus of a social goal

M = Mom; T = Teacher; C = Consultant; Sp Path = Speech and Language Pathologist

M:	…with the person once they get there.
Sp Path:	Like a game.
C:	Right. Still we are at the point right now where she is not particularly caring to play.
M:	Right.
C:	I almost wonder if we are going to need to look at some kind of reciprocal back and forth with a peer?
M:	And enjoy it!
C:	Right. We hope she will enjoy it.
T:	Yes.
M:	So like throwing a ball or passing a book back and forth.
C:	Right. So that she is engaging in some kind of back and forth activity, and we can't measure enjoyment but she is looking at the peer.
Sp Path:	I can't remember what the activity was, maybe dance but there were acouple of activities where she went and took kids' hands.
T:	I think you too (mom) were over by the table ,'cause I remember you were so excited by it and you mentioned it.
M:	She likes Ring around the Rosy.
Sp Path:	Yes, maybe it was some kind of motor activity.
T:	And scarves. She gets very motivated if we have those.
C:	Alright. So we need to figure out on this one how we can write a goal so it's very specific.. Those are really good activities, but may not necessarily be helpful for going back and forth.
M:	Right.
C:	So it may be that we just want her to engage in an activity for a certain number of minutes with a peer where she is……
Sp Path:	It's almost like you would have her to do some kind of physical play.
T:	Right.
Sp Path:	Where you just have another kid and you put a toy in there.
T:	But the attention isn't going to be on the person anymore.
C:	Right. Is she doing something interactive with kids now?
T:	We always share supplies. We take turns in circle. But when she has free time she just runs and explores her own thing.
M:	She can do it.
C:	But her preference, or her way of doing it is by herself, right? She really doesn't look much at the other child so it's really to define clearly what exactly we want her to do.
M:	She will take the figurine she is using and set it up on the VCR or move it along.
C:	Right. So there is interaction with objects. At home you see her doing more parallel play where she is using more materials, maybe there is some brief interactions but it's not really interactive or cooperative. At school she is really unaware of other children while doing her own activities. It sounds like you are wanting her to beplaying and interactive with other children. Is that right?
M:	Uh, huh.
C:	So what we want to think about is where at the end of the school year do we see her?
T:	Right, right.
M:	Here the kids in her class are having some of the same struggles she is. Her siblings, I've noticed, are starting to pull away a little more from her. But I direct them. I say, "Go in there," "Go do this," or "Go do that." So from whichever angle it's coming from at home, she is not being given a choice.
C:	Yes, this is work for her.
M:	So, I think the difference is not that they are giving her a choice, but the other children are having the same struggles as she is here.

Fig. 7.8 (continued)

M = Mom; T = Teacher; C = Consultant; Sp Path = Speech and Language Pathologist

C:	And that is an environmental challenge that we will have to talk about in the teaching plan. If there is a way for her to be with more social peers, like in her morning class.
T:	That would be something to observe in our classroom, more socialization.
C:	Maybe she could practice in your classroom and generalize to other peers in her morning class?
T:	Right. We could work that out.
C:	Perfect!
M:	So is that where we should bring in her morning teacher?
T:	That was my question. Is it possible for you to help us with the other environment?
C:	Oh, absolutely.
T:	I don't know if that needs to be noted because a lot of these skills are coming across in where we can't totally teach it in this environment, so she needs the dual placement.
C:	Right.
T:	She will interact at a sand table or water table briefly with guidance. It's just on her own she will probably walk away from the table.
C:	Well we would like her to do is do it with a peer, the peer doing all the prompting.
Sp Path:	Then it has got to be in the other environment.
C:	But she could practice it in this setting, right?
Sp Path:	Yes with us being the model.
T:	Right.
C:	She could practice with the adults then she could generalize with plans to the peer. That's just an example what it might actually look like. I'm sure you have lots of other ideas. I think playing with the ball is something she can do with a peer with you there doing the prompting at first.
Sp Path:	Right, Yes.
C:	But still she is learning the skill she needs which is to watch and to keep engaged.
Sp Path:	And we can do that here easily because there are a couple other ones in her class. We also have other kids that are pretty verbal and some in other classrooms that we can pull from to help.
Mom:	Is that something that could be beneficial to the other child though, too?
Sp Path:	Sure.
C:	Yes.
T:	Doing the same skills.
M:	Right, that's what I am wondering, if there is someone like that? And we could sit down and talk to her morning teacher, too, about it. And purposefully target other children than just her brother.
T:	Right.
Sp Path:	'Cause she is comfortable with that.
M:	Very much so.
T:	I think her brother gives her what she wants. She has fresh peers in this class that age appropriately will say "No," so it changes her scheme of what she is used.
M:	So maybe we could ask if there is someone in her class in the other school that we could pull in.
C:	Ok let's see if we can do that with the conditions given, what's the condition? That she has sociable peers? This is what we want her to be doing by the end of the year. Is this during free play, structure or unstructured time?
T:	Well that is one of her goals. We want her to find a friend and request play.
Sp Path:	So during a structured activity she will initiate the play with a friend. But that's not the end goal probably.

Fig. 7.8 (continued)

M = Mom; T = Teacher; C = Consultant; Sp Path = Speech and Language Pathologist

C: I guess I would like to see her engage in some kind of reciprocal back and forth for
            a certain amount of time or certain number of exchanges so we are keeping her on
            target. Like the ball.

Sp Path: Right.

T: Yes. I keep going back to the ball 'cause often when she knows we are going outside
            and she will ask for the beach ball or ask for the princess ball. She will take it outside
            and she will kind of kick it somewhere and then she is done. That might be a good start
            - where it's something she has been interested in and show her how to keep it up.

C: Right and where she is going back and forth so she is going to engage in "X" num-
            ber of reciprocal interactions with a peer.

M: Exchanges.

C: And an exchange is one back and forth interchange. That's how we can define one
            exchange.

T: Is that prompting or a person prompting?

C: It's going to have to be structured. The prompting is part of the condition. But again
            think about the end of the year where you would like to see her. So it could be peer
            prompting with adults out of it.

M: That's what I was going to suggest, is it be a peer rather than an adult.

C: Ok, so given a structured play activity She will.... What?

Sp Path: Reciprocal exchanges.

C: And how many?

Sp Path: And is this the end of the year?

C: Yes.

T: The ultimate target.

C: Play through how many exchanges?

M: How do you put a number on that?

Sp Path: I mean at least 4.

T: Maybe 3 to 4. I was going to say once you hit 3...

Sp Path: So it could be a ball activity, some kind of game activity.

C: So we are going to play through 4 exchanges and should we say...

M: That just goes back to her attention span.

C: You know if we get to this we just keep going, expect more.

M: Extend it.

C: And how many play activities? I think we should probably put a number on it.
            Because we could say she has met it if we do it with the ball only. So how many
            different play activities?

M: Is three a good number - Three or four. ?

C: Three different structured play activities?

M: Just trying to think of things she likes, her little people or weebles or a game.

T: Games would be easy to share.

Sp Path: It's got to be where the other kid needed to complete the activity.

C: Why?

Sp Path: It's like what kind of activity and the other child is needed to complete it, whether
            it's roll a ball.

C: Or you just set it up that you need to exchange it at least four times. You only have
            one item and they need to share it.

Sp Path: Mmm.

C: And she is interested in whatever it is. And they are working on or playing with
            something together.

M = Mom; T = Teacher; C = Consultant; Sp Path = Speech and Language Pathologist

Fig. 7.8 (continued)

M = Mom; T = Teacher; C = Consultant; Sp Path = Speech and Language Pathologist	
T:	One glue stick, or something like that.
C:	And I guess, you know we may have to go to what we mean by reciprocal I think we know ,but we are really looking at trying to get her to look at the child. I'll write something and put a little note in here so we are sure we are all clear on what that means.
T:	Yes.
Sp Path:	Is it physical or touching the child?
C:	Right, yes. Ok, how often will we want to see her do that? The question is how many times will she have opportunities to play the three different activities during the week?
Sp Path:	Do we have to do all three schemes or are we just doing one scheme?
C:	That's what we will have to decide? You just decide what makes sense.
M:	Or is three like an ultimate goal? That's not three daily is it? That seems overwhelming.
T:	I would hope we could give her the opportunity to practice at least two schemes a day
C:	It's whatever you want to do or at least twice a day with at least two different objects. We know for her to learn we want her to have as many opportunities as possible, so two times a day and you keep data what … weekly?
T:	Daily, we try to write down what we have done.
C:	You do everyday?
T:	What the result is.
C:	Okay, two times a day. Is that clear enough?
T:	Should we say on 80 % on the collection opportunities?
C:	Ok? Just so we are clear. The way this is worded we are cancelling out where she is doing the dancing kind of thing 'cause it's not really reciprocal.
Sp Path:	Well with one scarf they could take turns with one scarf.
C:	That's right.
T:	That's true.
C:	Yes, we could make it a reciprocal.
Sp Path:	Yes, with dance.
C:	The measurable social goal then is "Given 3 different structured play activities (e.g., ball, scarf dancing), she will play through four exchanges with a peer (peer prompts only) twice a day for two activities by the end of the school year." We will write the teaching plan when we have the other two goals.We have an hour and a half left.

Fig. 7.8 (continued)

Write Measurable IEP Objectives for the Consensus Areas

Once the team has gained consensus on at least three skills, write the skill as an IEP objective that is measurable and observable on the *Develop COMPASS Teaching Plan: Environmental Support Form* provided in the COMPASS Consultation Training Packet. Be sure to describe the level of prompting that will be applied. If there is no prompting (other than the use of visual supports or some other environmental support), then it is assumed that the child will complete the skill independently. Chapter 5 has more details on high quality IEPs of students with autism and how to write measurable objectives. Also, list the criterion for success or how many times the child must be able to perform the skill in order to state that the objective was met. Finally, the skill must be specific and observable. If a stranger can read the objective and be able to observe the skill with clarity of how it "looks," know when the skill is achieved, and know what conditions under which the skill is performed, then the IEP objective is measurable and observable. Figure 7.8 illustrates a discussion of developing consensus on a social goal.

Develop COMPASS Teaching Plans for Each Measurable Objective

For each measurable objective, the COMPASS teaching plans are developed. This is often the task that takes the most time during the consultation. It is especially important that the consultant does not do the work for the team, but rather ask the team for input as well as provide guiding questions. To be effective in this process, an understanding of autism and use of the salient information provided during the review of the COMPASS Challenges and Supports forms, as well as the ability to use Socratic questioning techniques to facilitate the team's input into each of the four components that make up the teaching plan is necessary. The Socratic inter-viewing technique is based on the principle that although the consultant may know the answer to a question, she asks questions as if she does not know in order to guide the parent and teacher to the answer. This allows parents and teachers to have the experience of reaching the answers by themselves. The use of the Socratic inter-viewing method broadens views by helping parents and teachers discover all the possible aspects involved in answering a question. It empowers participants by expanding their personal sense of control and understanding of the issues and ques-tions at hand. The COMPASS consultation is a process of teaching and learning between all the participants. The team is thinking logically together in order to cre-ate new meanings and new knowledge shared among all the participants. This pro-cess requires much self-reflection and self-scrutiny on the side of the consultant, the parent, and the teacher. An authentic exchange of the child's environmental chal-lenges and the supports necessary to counter the challenges results in better plans when self-scrutiny can occur within a trusting and collaborative relationship. It is critical for the consultant to be nonjudgmental and to use active listening skills dur-ing this aspect of the consultation. Figure 7.9 illustrates a discussion on the personal and environmental challenges and supports necessary to consider for a student who is learning to take turns.

Following the discussion of the personal and environmental challenges and sup-ports for each skill, the other activities outlined in Table 7.5 are conducted. Provided in Fig. 7.10 is an example of a completed description of the personal and environ-mental challenges and supports based on the discussion provided in Fig. 7.9.

After discussion of the relationship between the objective and the personal challenges and supports that will hinder or facilitate learning, the next step is to complete the COMPASS Teaching Plan: Environmental Supports Form and the activities described in Table 7.6. Attend to specific details of what evidence base

M = Mom; T = Teacher; C = Consultant; Sp Path = Speech and Language Pathologist	
C:	Okay, so what we want to do is go back to the social goal [the goal is when given three different structured play activities (e.g., ball, scarf dancing), she will play through four exchanges with a peer twice a day for two activities for 80% of opportunities by the end of the school year]. What are the personal challenges that she has for reaching this goal - the kind of things that we know are going to have to be balanced with our teaching strategies? What are the challenges for her to accomplish this skill?
T:	Motivation.
C:	Okay
Sp Path:	And interest.
M:	That's going to apply for every one of these. Distractions will apply to others.
Sp Path:	Yes, distractions.
M:	You know some of that could be hereditary. I get distracted lots of times.
C:	We all have some of this.
	[Laughter from the group]
C:	And her eye contact problem, just not looking at the other kids. So the distractions are everything in the environment that happen to be there. The challenges in the classroom in the afternoon are finding sociable peers.
T:	That's what I was thinking to say. We don't have sociable peers. They don't have her interests.
C:	Right.
T:	We can try to set her up with peers.
Sp Path:	Yes I think we can.
M:	Are there other peers? I mean I don't want to disrupt her class.
Sp Path:	In her class there are a couple of girls who are verbal who could interact with her.
C:	Good. What are some personal supports that she has within herself?
T:	She's social. That she does enjoy different play options.
C:	Right.
T:	She has the idea when we say go play what that means.
M:	She knows what she wants.
T:	Right and she does act appropriately. She won't hit someone.
M:	Mostly…
C:	Well and a personal support is her reading. Then an environmental support she has is all of you working together.
M:	And her brothers and sisters.
C:	Yes, and she has visual supports. Just lots of things are in place and we want her to function in natural environments.
M:	Yes.
C:	So the distractions are just part of being in those environments.

Fig. 7.9 Excerpt on discussion of personal and environmental challenges and supports for social skills teaching plan

Table 7.5 COMPASS components to consider for personalized teaching plans

For all three objectives, use the COMPASS balance between challenges and supports form to:
Write each prioritized concern as a measurable objective
Identify personal and environmental challenges that may interfere with learning this skill
Identify personal and environmental supports for learning this skill

IEP Objective	Personal Challenges	Environmental Challenges	Personal Supports	Environmental Supports
Given 3 different structured play activities (e.g., ball, scarf dancing), she will play through 4 exchanges with a peer twice a day for two activities for 80% of opportunities by the end of the school year.	• Lack of motivation • Easily distracted • Poor use of eye contact and limited joint attention	• Access to sociable peers in afternoon • Lack of "trained" peer • Distracting environments	• Enjoys different play objects/toys • Has idea of "go play" • Knows what she wants–has preferences of certain objects • Acts appropriately – doesn't hit others • Willing to be close to others • Learns by watching • Reads	• Identify sociable peers and teach them to play with her and coach her • Include her sociable siblings in purposeful play • Use visual supports – videos and models to help teach concepts • Use social story • Provide lots of opportunities to practice • See teaching plan for specific details

Fig. 7.10 COMPASS balance between challenges and supports

practice will be considered in teaching the skill (see handout in Forms section of this chapter), what activities you will use or need to develop to teach the skill, what materials will be necessary to use or to create, who, where, and when instruction will occur, and how data will be collected. As this information is being considered, be sure to include the child's strengths and preferences in planning. Next, plan what cues will be used and how many; also decide on how reinforcement will be applied for correct and incorrect responses. For incorrect responses, because persons with autism often have a delay in processing information, it is important to allow at least 3–5 s before attempting to prompt the child again. It is also important to consider the types of prompts you will use and to start with the least invasive prompt before moving to a more restrictive prompt. More discussion of prompting is available online from the National Professional Development Center on Autism Spectrum Disorders and also in the next chapter. Table 7.6 describes essential details for planning effective teaching plans as well as offers questions to consider for the teaching plans. Figure 7.11 illustrates a discussion of an actual teaching plan, and Fig. 7.12 shows the completed teaching plan based on the discussion. Both of these examples are based on the IEP objective described in Fig. 7.10. After the teaching plans are written, provide a copy of the handwritten objectives and teaching plans to the members.

Table 7.6 Guide to developing a teaching plan

Using a COMPASS Teaching Plan: Environmental Supports Form (one form for each skill)…

a. Review the evidence based practices that are relevant for the skill

b. Identify the activities and materials to be used for teaching the skill

    Question: What are the child's strengths and skill preferences?

C. Identify additional supports to maximize competence

    Questions: What visuals are best?

             What models will be useful (objects, other children)?

             What place will maximize attention?

C. Identify the initial cue

    Questions: Will cue(s) be visual, verbal, gestural, or a combination?

             How close in proximity will the person be when giving the cue?

             What eye level would be optimal?

             Who will give the cue?

             How many prompts will be given as part of the initial cue?

             How long will you wait between prompts?

D. Identify the reinforcement that will be used for correct behavior and how it will be delivered

E. Identify how you will respond to incorrect responses

F. Identify how often the skill needs to be worked on

G. Identify how and when data will be kept, how often it will be collected, and who is responsible to collect it

H. Identify who will work on the skill

M = Mom; T = Teacher; C = Consultant; Sp Path = Speech and Language Pathologist

C: Okay, with the social goal we talked about exactly how are we going to start to teach the skill? What are the steps we want to have in place? We talked about first identifying peers. And this will help us to think about the teaching plan. So we've identified sociable peers and some activities that are going to be motivating to her. On your handout on resources for teachers there some nice websites on how to identify and train peers - like how to get her attention and what to do if she walks away. Things like that.

T: And preschoolers are good at this

M: They are really good at this. Well and if there is stuff to train peers that would be huge for us at home.

C: You want to have kids who can pay attention for at least 5 - 10 minutes. Look under peer mediated instruction.

Sp Path: We might have to get 1st graders.

C: Yes, but preschoolers can do this.

T: So there would be training for them. Like practice?

C: Oh, yes.

T: Um, ok and then we need to do what else?

C: Define the situations.

Sp Path: Maybe one can be sharing.

M: She loves music.

T: They could take turns with musical instruments.

Sp Path: They can switch.

T: See I think she can do that but I don't see her doing it on her own.

C: No this is work for her, learning to play is work for her.

M: Yes.

T: So this will be like we have done turn taking. She can with the adult.

Fig. 7.11 Excerpt on discussion of teaching plan for social skills

M = Mom; T = Teacher; C = Consultant; Sp Path = Speech and Language Pathologist	
Sp Path:	Like she likes matching wands, maybe there is a special wand. We don't say in here… does she say 'my turn' or how does she get the turn?
M:	Well, no 'cause we left it more open if it is ball play or the scarves.
T:	So since she is capable of turn taking she is very capable of playing the "my turn" game.
C:	Yes.
M:	Hm.
Sp Path:	But maybe if we structure it as not necessarily it's my turn with the red scarf, but this is the way it works and so dances with the blue scarf.
T:	And then switch. We play with tapping sticks. You hand your sticks to your neighbor.
C:	Right.
Sp Path:	Maybe it's easier to start with passing something, then work up to different colors.
M:	Yes.
C:	Maybe it addresses that this is the way we play the game more than we are going to take turns.
T:	Right.
C:	I think, too, that the activities that work best are those where there is nice engagement between the two children. There is the reciprocal, back and forth interaction.
Sp Path:	Well you can't do "Row Row Your Boat" unless you both do it, can you?
T:	I don't really see that as reciprocal.
M:	It's not.
Sp Path:	It's engaging.
C:	Yes, It's engaging.
T:	What about if we are playing "Bob the Builder" with a peg builder and take turns with the hammer?
C:	Yes.
T:	Until we get them all done.
C:	Yes.
T:	My turn, your turn back and forth. Let's finish the whole thing.
C:	So we are all working on the same thing.
T:	Right.
M:	Yes. Sometimes it's hard for her to keep doing it. She likes "Duck duck goose." Does that count as reciprocal?
C:	Reciprocal, joint attention.
M:	Hmm.
T:	And that's really important for her.
M:	Yes.
Sp Path:	That's a group one. That's what I see is missing.
T:	She doesn't do that.
M:	She does at home. I mean if she wants too.
T:	Right, right. And it's probably here 'cause we don't have enough kids for her to engage with a group.
M:	I'm sure in the morning program there are multiple kinds of things they do in groups.
C:	Okay. So we just have identified some of the activities after we have an activity all set up then what do we do? What are some strategies we are going to use to teach her?
Sp Path:	Well go to verbal, "Whose turn is it?" We could use a visual for "my turn" where she actually has to get a card with words.
T:	Says, "It's my turn."
M:	Yes.
T:	Yes. It goes back and forth between the kids.
C:	If you made a video of doing this and showed it to her, would she watch it?
M:	Oh, that would be good.
C:	Video modeling for her.
T:	I found even when we try to do the ball exchange - physically. Yes, I mean if we are rolling the ball for her.

Fig. 7.11 (continued)

M = Mom; T = Teacher; C = Consultant; Sp Path = Speech and Language Pathologist
M: If we are just standing there. She is in space. And seeing her brothers and sisters doing it and watching it helps.
C: We always want her to see herself doing it positively or correctly. Watching others model the skill helps her too.
M: Another activity we go do is face painting or something on each other.
T: Hmm.
M: Doing something like putting stickers on each other. So it's more of a natural.
T: Fun. Princess stickers.
M: She likes make up or stickers on her nose. Her make-up! It's more like my make-up.
C: Reciprocal play, that's good. Let's look at what we have so far for the teaching plan. Before the first coaching you will have time to think about these and try some activities and strategies out. Then we will go from there. So far we have [the consultant reviews the teaching plan in Figure 7.12].

Fig. 7.11 (continued)

Teaching Methods	Who/Where/When
• Identify sociable peers and coach them on how to play with her (see online resources for teachers from **NPDC** and **OCALI** on peer mediated instruction) • Set up situations using objects and activities that interest her (musical instruments, scarves, wand, stickers on face) (see online resources for teachers from **NPDC** and **OCALI** on pivotal response training) • Provide direct instruction with her on "taking turns" using a social story and role-playing with an adult and peer • For activities that involve turn-taking, use a "My turn" card • Make a video of children taking turns and of herself taking turns (see online resources for teachers from **NPDC** on video self modeling) • Provide praise/reinforcement for taking turns with peers	With peers in the morning and afternoon classrooms twice a day
	Materials Turn taking activities Visual script of "My turn" Social story on taking turns
	Data System Activity based data sheet completed two times a week

Fig. 7.12 Teaching plan for social skills based on the IEP objective in Fig. 7.10

Summarize and Close

You will discuss follow-up activities and outline next steps:

1. Ask the team to update the student's IEP within 3 weeks to address any changes and to assure that COMPASS information and prioritized objectives are included
2. Set up the first coaching session with the teacher and parent. Caregivers may not be able to attend, but remind them that they will receive a report from the coaching session
3. Provide team members a COMPASS Consultation Satisfaction Questionnaire to complete as well as a COMPASS Consultation Fidelity Checklist. This checklist can be returned by mail or fax if necessary
4. Provide a written summary of the objectives and teaching plans to teachers and parents within 1 week

Appendix A   Instructions for Completing Step B of COMPASS Consultation Action Plan

In the following section, we provide you with the forms and handouts you will need to conduct a COMPASS consultation. Instructions for the forms are given below.

A. Read over the COMPASS Consultation Protocol and have a copy available for yourself during the consultation, which includes instructions for completing the following steps:

 1. Sign in and introductions
 2. Explanation of COMPASS
 3. Explanation of purpose/outcomes of COMPASS consultation
 4. Overview of best practices
 5. Gain consensus

    a. Review COMPASS Consultation Joint Summary
    b. Identify a social skill, communication skill, and learning skill objective
    c. Agree on top three concerns

 6. Develop teaching plan for each concern
 7. Summarize and close

B. At the start of the consultation, have all participants complete the COMPASS Sign-in Sheet.
C. Provide copies of the COMPASS Consultation Training Packet to each participant, which includes the following items:

 1. Purpose/outcomes of COMPASS consultation
 2. Illustration of iceberg
 3. Overview of Best Practices for Individualized Education Plans (IEP) for Young Students with ASD
 4. Prioritize teacher and caregiver goals and write measurable objectives
 5. Develop compass teaching plan: Environmental supports (make three copies of this form or as many needed for each skill)
 6. COMPASS Consultation Satisfaction Questionnaire
 7. COMPASS Consultation Fidelity Checklist

D. Follow the COMPASS consultation protocol for each activity.

Appendix B   Abridged Protocol for Step B of the COMPASS Consultation Action Plan

Discuss COMPASS Consultation Training Packet

Introductions and Sign In

Below is a sample introduction script. Please note: It is important that you apply your own style of interaction and use your own words, as an important attribute of an effective consultant is authenticity.

> You know (student's name) better than I do. By working collaboratively using all of our knowledge and expertise, we can enhance (name's) response to his/her educational program. You have already provided us with a wealth of information about (student's name), which we will use today as we all plan together. I am here as a facilitator. I will be using the COMPASS Model to better understand (student's name) and develop a personalized program based on current best practices and your priorities for (student's name).

Explanation of COMPASS

Hand out the COMPASS Consultation Training Packet and refer to the Balance.

Sample script:
Our goal is to enhance (student's name) competence by considering how to balance personal and environmental challenges with personal and environmental supports. The challenges are the risk factors that may keep a student from learning. These include those within the child (personal factors) and those that the environment creates for the student (environmental factors). The supports are protective factors and include personnel strengths and interests and environmental supports such as teaching strategies and various accommodations. In order for a student to be successful there must be enough on the support side to balance the risks.

Explanation of Purpose/Outcomes of COMPASS Consultation

Distribute and discuss the *Purpose/Outcomes of COMPASS Consultation* handout, which is located later in this chapter. For your convenience, we also provide the content of the handout below.

Purpose/Outcomes of COMPASS Consultation

1. Enhance parent–teacher collaboration in order to provide a holistic assessment of the student's current functioning, learning, and needs.
2. Provide a process to reach consensus on recommendations for an individualized educational program including specific positive, individualized teaching strategies.

3. Write three measurable objectives from prioritized goals and develop specific teaching strategies for these.
4. Enhance purposeful and active student engagement in learning.

Overview of Best Practices

Distribute and discuss the *Overview of Best Practices for IEP for Young Students with ASD* handout, which is located later in this chapter. For your convenience, we also provide the content of the handout below.

Overview of Best Practices

The IEP should be the method utilized to identify objectives and strategies to achieve educational objectives. The educational objectives should include the growth of:

* Social skills to improve involvement in school, family and community activities (e.g., parallel and interactive play with family members and peers).
* Expressive verbal language, receptive language, and nonverbal communication skills.
* A symbolic communication system that is functional.
* Engagement and flexibility in tasks and play that are developmentally appropriate. This should also include the ability to be aware of the environment and respond to appropriate motivational systems.
* Fine and gross motor skills to be utilized when engaging in age appropriate activities.
* Cognitive or thinking skills, which include academic skills, basic concepts, and symbolic play. Replacement of problem behavior with more conventional or appropriate behavior.
* Behaviors that are the foundation to success in a regular classroom (following instructions, completing a task) and independent organizational skills.

Discuss the COMPASS Consultation Joint Summary

Review summary information from *Consultation Summary Packet* (allow about 60 min). By reviewing the summarized information with the teacher and parent, insight will be gained to help understand how the model works, assessing accuracy of information and whether additional information is necessary.

Identify and Come to a Consensus on the Top Three Concerns

Identify top three concerns: Consolidate and emphasize social, communication, and work skills using COMPASS Summary of Concerns. The caregiver and teacher agree on top three concerns within each domain with assistance from the consultant who facilitates prioritizing a social skill, a communication skill, and a learning or work skill.

Develop COMPASS Teaching Plans for Each Measurable Objective

For all three objectives, use the COMPASS Balance Between Challenges and Supports Form to:

- Write each prioritized concern as a measurable objective
- Identify personal and environmental challenges that may interfere with learning this skill
- Identify personal and environmental supports for learning this skill

Using a COMPASS Teaching Plan: Environmental Supports Form (one form for each skill), identify:

- Teaching methods (see Tables 7.5 and 7.6 and Explanation of Evidence Based Practices in Forms section)
- Materials
- Who will be responsible for teaching the objective, where the teaching will occur, and when
- The data system

Summarize and Close

Describe next steps:

- IEP Development Meeting within 3 weeks to address any changes and to assure that COMPASS information and prioritized objectives are included.
- Coaching with teacher and caregiver, if possible, will occur every 4–6 weeks.

Allow 10 min to complete follow-up forms, or ask participants to complete these later and send to you within 3 days:

- Complete COMPASS Consultation Satisfaction Questionnaire.
- Complete COMPASS Consultation Fidelity Checklist.

Give written or printed copy of each objective to the participants if possible.

Consultant provides a written summary of teaching plans for each objective to teachers and caregivers within 1 week.

Appendix C   COMPASS Consultation Sign-In Sheet

Please print:

Student's Name: _____ Consultation Date:_____

Name of School: _____

Parent's Name: _____

Caregiver's Name: _____

Special Education Teacher's Name: _____

All caregivers, teachers, and others who interact regularly with the student and who will participate in the COMPASS consultation need to complete the following:

Name	Title	Average number of hours per week with child

Appendix D   COMPASS Consultation Training Packet

Created for (student's name):_____ Date:_____

Caregiver's name:_____

Teacher's name:_____

Consultant's name:_____

COMPASS: Providing Direction

A Collaborative Model
for Promoting
Competence and Success
for Persons with
Autism Spectrum Disorder

Balancing Challenges and Supports

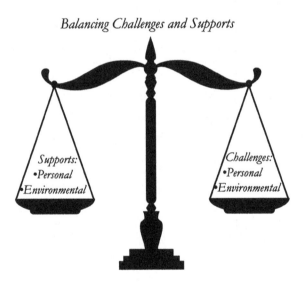

1. Enhance caregiver–teacher collaboration in order to provide a holistic assessment of the student's current functioning, learning, and needs.
2. Provide a process to reach consensus on recommendations for an individualized educational program including specific positive, individualized teaching strategies.
3. Write three measurable objectives from prioritized goals within the social, communication, and learning or work-skill domains. Develop specific teaching strategies for each.
4. Enhance purposeful and active student engagement in learning.
5. Review the Overview of Best Practices for IEP for Young Students with ASD

Iceberg

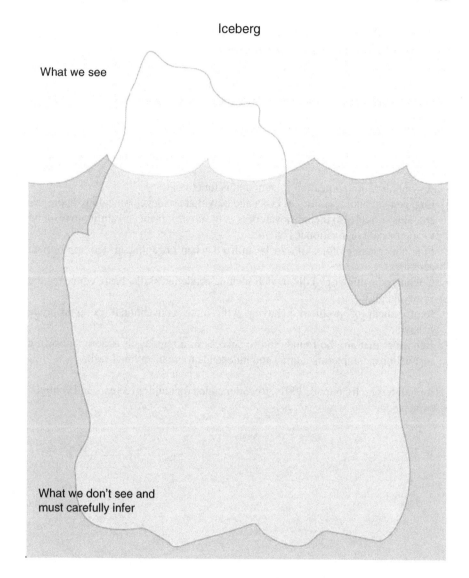

What we see

What we don't see and
must carefully infer

Overview of Best Practices for Individualized Education Plan (IEP) for Students with ASD

The IEP should be the method utilized to obtain planning and educational objectives. The educational objectives should include the growth of the following:

- Social skills to improve involvement in school, family, and community activities (e.g., parallel and interactive play with family members and peers).
- Expressive verbal language, receptive language, and nonverbal communication skills.
- A symbolic communication system that is functional.
- Engagement and flexibility in tasks and play that are developmentally appropriate. This should also include awareness of the environment and ability to respond to appropriate motivational systems.
- Fine and gross motor skills to be utilized when engaging in age appropriate activities.
- Cognitive or thinking skills, which include academic skills, basic concepts and symbolic play.
- Replacement of problem behavior with more conventional or appropriate behavior.
- Behaviors that are the foundation to success in a regular classroom (following instructions, completing a task) and independent organizational skills.

(National Research Council, 2001). Recommended for children 8 years and younger, www.nap.edu.

Prioritize Teacher and Caregiver Goals and Write Measurable Objectives

Student's Name: _____ Teacher's Name: _____

Social and Play Skills

Concern/Skill:
Measurable Objective:

Communication Skills

Concern/Skill:
Measurable Objective:

Learning Skills

Concern/Skill:
Measurable Objective:

Compass Balance Between Challenges and Supports

IEP objective	Personal challenges	Environmental challenges	Personal supports	Environmental supports

COMPASS Teaching Plan: Environmental Supports

Student's Name: _____ Teacher's Name: _____

Teaching Objective:

Teaching Methods	Who/Where/When
	Materials
	Data System

COMPASS Consultation Satisfaction Questionnaire

Student's Name: _____Your Relationship to Child:_____

Your Name: _____ Date:_____

Directions: Rate your experience with the COMPASS program, with "1" meaning "Strongly Disagree" and "4" meaning "Strongly Agree." For questions that are not applicable, select "NA."

		Strongly disagree			Strongly agree	
1.	I felt involved during the consultation and able to express my views.	1	2	3	4	NA
2.	The consultant's communication skills were effective.	1	2	3	4	NA
3.	The consultant listened to what I had to say.	1	2	3	4	NA
4.	The consultant was knowledgeable about ASD.	1	2	3	4	NA
5.	The consultant was able to adapt recommendations/suggestions based on my particular situation/classroom.	1	2	3	4	NA
6.	The consultation made me think differently about the cause(s) of my child's behavior.	1	2	3	4	NA
7.	The consultant gave me new information about ways my child/student learns.	1	2	3	4	NA
8.	I gained a better understanding of how ASD affects my child/student.	1	2	3	4	NA
9.	I learned a useful way to problem-solve as a team on behalf of my child/student.	1	2	3	4	NA
10.	I gained a better understanding of other team members' points of view.	1	2	3	4	NA
11.	I felt team members gained a better understanding of my point of view.	1	2	3	4	NA
12.	I gained a better understanding of specific teaching strategies for my child/student.	1	2	3	4	NA
13.	I gained a better understanding about what is needed in my child's/student's IEP.	1	2	3	4	NA
14.	I gained a more holistic understanding of my child/student (at home, school, community).	1	2	3	4	NA
15.	A more holistic understanding of my child/student is useful for understanding why she/he does what she/he does.	1	2	3	4	NA
16.	The consultation was helpful in gaining consensus on my child's/student's IEP goals.	1	2	3	4	NA
17.	This consultation was helpful in gaining consensus on specific teaching strategies.	1	2	3	4	NA
18.	I will change some ways I interact with my child/student based on information from this consultation.	1	2	3	4	NA
19.	My child's/student's IEP will change based on this consultation.	1	2	3	4	NA
20.	The problem-solving process used in this consultation will be helpful with future work with my child/student.	1	2	3	4	NA

		Strongly disagree				Strongly agree
21.	I feel comfortable in using the COMPASS problem-solving process on my own with my school team to develop/monitor my child's/student's program.	1	2	3	4	NA
22.	I will update the information concerning my child's/student's challenges/supports on an ongoing basis.	1	2	3	4	NA
23.	The time allotted for this consultation was adequate.	1	2	3	4	NA
24.	Overall, I feel that the consultation was collaborative.	1	2	3	4	NA
25.	Overall, I am satisfied with the consultation.	1	2	3	4	NA

26. What was most helpful about the consultation?

27. What would you recommend to improve the consultation?

28. What supports do you need in order to implement the ideas shared in the consultation?

29. What barriers do you foresee in being able to implement the ideas shared in the consultation?

Thank you!

COMPASS Consultation Fidelity Checklist

Instructions: Below are the components of the COMPASS consultation. Check the following boxes for the elements that occurred during the consultation.

1. The COMPASS consultation comprises a multidisciplinary team defined by:

- ❑ teacher and parents attend meeting
- ❑ other personnel who interact regularly with student attend meeting

2. COMPASS is collaborative as defined by:

- ❑ goals include those suggested from home and family
- ❑ planning for the student's program is based on input from all participants
- ❑ each member contributes ideas for teaching the goals

3. The COMPASS consultation process incorporates the following:

- ❑ checklists that are used to help organize information, identify student's needs, and solicit input from all members
- ❑ facilitated guidance and structure from the consultant
- ❑ a picture of the student at home, in the community, and at school

4. IEP goals that came from the COMPASS consultation are the following:

- ❑ described in clear behavioral terms
- ❑ measurable and observable

5. COMPASS consultation results in a teaching plan that:

- ❑ identifies at least three priority concerns
- ❑ prioritizes concerns that relate to home, community and school
- ❑ identifies specific skills that the student must learn in order to accomplish each of the priority concerns
- ❑ links the specific teaching strategies to each identified skill

6. The teaching strategies described in the COMPASS plan:

- ❑ are developed AFTER goals are generated
- ❑ are individualized for the student and the goal
- ❑ are described in behavioral terms

7. Team believes that the student's ability to learn is based on environmental and student factors:

- ❑ there was a discussion of specific environmental factors for each goal
- ❑ the philosophy of the environment as an important factor in determining student progress is discussed
- ❑ team completes and discusses COMPASS forms on student's strengths/challenges and environment's strengths/challenges

8. COMPASS results in members having a broader understanding of the student:

- ❑ family members report that they have a better perspective on school issues
- ❑ teachers report that they have a better perspective on home and community issues

9. COMPASS consultation results in proactive problem solving:

- ❑ interactive problem solving is implemented by team members providing input and ideas
- ❑ specific problems for implementation and solutions are identified
- ❑ members learn a framework for problem solving that can be used again by individual team members when needed

Evidence-Based Online Resources for Teachers

Direct links to each of these Web sites are available at http://www.ukautism.org/onlineresources.php. We will update our Web site regularly with any changes in the URLs. Visit this Web site for the latest links and for new suggested Web sites.

Recommended Web sites

All resources in this section are available from the following recommended Web sites. Each domain below lists the Web site name:

- Autism Services Research Group: COMPASS Series, http://www.ukautism.org/
- Interactive Collaborative Autism Network (ICAN), http://www.autismnetwork.org/
- National Professional Development Center on Autism Spectrum Disorders (NPDC), http://autismpdc.fpg.unc.edu/
- Ohio Center for Autism and Low Incidence: Autism Internet Modules (OCALI) All modules have a video and requires an account to be set up with a login and password, http://www.autisminternetmodules.org/

Social (See Recommended Web sites for Specific URL)

- COMPASS Series: Early Social Skills
- COMPASS Series: Teaching Social Interaction and Play within a Peer Group
- ICAN: Social Interventions (peer-mediated instruction, social stories)
- NPDC & OCALI: Peer-Mediated Instruction and Intervention
- NPDC: Social Narratives
- NPDC: Social Skills Groups
- NPDC: Video Modeling

Communication

- ICAN: Communication Interventions (augmentative and alternative communication; naturalistic language strategies; joint action routines; picture exchange communication system)
- NPDC: Session 7 Foundations of Communication and Social Intervention
- NPDC: Picture Exchange Communication System & OCALI PECS
- NPDC: Functional Communication Training
- NPDC: Speech Generating Devices/VOCA
- NPDC & OCALI: Naturalistic Intervention
- NPDC & OCALI: Pivotal Response Training
- OCALI: Computer Aided Instruction (follow autism in the classroom and at home links)

Learning Skills

- NPDC: Session 6 Instructional strategies and learning environments
- NPDC & OCALI: Self-Management
- NPDC & OCALI: Visual Supports
- NPDC & OCALI: Structured Work Systems
- OCALI: Structured Teaching

Behavior

- COMPASS Series: Behavior Management
- COMPASS Series: Relaxation/Calming
- ICAN: Behavioral Interventions
- NPDC: Session 8 Promoting positive behavior and reducing interfering behaviors
- NPDC: Extinction
- NPDC & OCALI: Antecedent-Based Intervention
- NPDC: Differential Reinforcement
- NPDC: Functional Behavior Assessment
- NPDC & OCALI: Response Interruption/Redirection

Self-help/Adaptive

- COMPASS Series: Toilet Training
- COMPASS Series: Constipation in Children with Autism
- COMPASS Series: Helping Your Child Sleep Better

General

- COMPASS Series: Elements of Effective Programs
- COMPASS Series: Understanding Death
- COMPASS Series: Visual Supports
- ICAN: Environmental Interventions
- NPDC & OCALI: Time Delay
- NPDC: Prompting
- NPDC & OCALI: Reinforcement

Chapter 8
From Consultation to Coaching: Implementing Plans and Monitoring Progress

Overview: This chapter covers the essential components of teacher coaching. The importance of follow-up sessions from the initial COMPASS consultation is described and coaching is defined. Also provided are practical forms and a coaching protocol. The primary outcome measure of a COMPASS consultation is described, and instructions are provided for developing the Goal Attainment Scale Form.

In this chapter, we describe the following:

1. The concept of coaching and how it differs from consultation.
2. The necessity of coaching sessions after consultation.
3. Intervention fidelity and its relationship to consultation outcomes.
4. The skills needed by a COMPASS coach.
5. The COMPASS Coaching Protocol and how to write and use the Goal Attainment Scale (GAS) Form to monitor student progress.
6. How to determine when to end the consultation process.

In this chapter, we outline what happens during a COMPASS coaching session. Coaching occurs after the completion of Steps A and B of the COMPASS Consultation Action Plan, which are covered in Chaps. 6 and 7.

What Is Coaching?

How is coaching different from consultation? Up to this point, we have referred to our intervention as a consultation program planning framework. Whereas consultation is an activity that sets the goals and plans the teaching strategies, coaching is the term used to describe the vehicle that puts the plans into practice. The terms consultant and coach are used interchangeably because it is assumed they are the same person who works with the same teacher, parent, and child. But there are some differences in the terms worth noting. Consultation has a strong history in mental health services and dates back more than 60 years. It occurs with a focus on the

L.A. Ruble et al., *Collaborative Model for Promoting Competence and Success for Students with ASD*, DOI 10.1007/978-1-4614-2332-4_8, © Springer Science+Business Media, LLC 2012

context of the classroom and involves all aspects of knowledge and skill transfer that is bidirectional in its focus on plan implementation. The coach and the teacher are partners who are engaged in a shared activity with a common goal. In summary, consultation serves to set the goals and plan the strategies, and coaching helps put the plans into practice. In COMPASS, the consultation is used to develop the teaching plans, and the subsequent activity of coaching helps put into practice the teaching plans developed during the consultation. The coaching follow-up sessions are designed to assist the teacher in evaluating the student's progress, evaluate the teaching strategies, model teaching strategies, and assist the teacher in performance feedback. Coaching sessions are necessary to ensure (or assure) that the teacher has the tools to adequately individualize instruction so that the student makes progress.

Coaching has become notable as a means to assist teachers in the hands-on application of skill. It was first described in the 1980s by Joyce and Showers (1983) as the means to transfer new skills and understandings within the teacher's own instructional setting. Coaching for application is an even more specific term and refers to direct hands-on, in-classroom assistance with the transfer of the skills and strategies to the classroom. Coaching refers to a formal relationship between a teacher and a coach. The COMPASS coach has expertise not only in autism but also in methods designed to assist the teacher in improving his or her teaching outcomes for students with autism. Both consultation and coaching are time-limited activities that can occur throughout a school year or over many years. The coach and the teacher set goals for the implementation of teaching plans that are mutually defined, and reflective action takes place during the coaching activity. Assessment is used to guide formal and informal feedback to teachers about their performance as related to the student's progress. Coaching is most commonly done face-to-face. However, in rural areas or areas where travel is difficult or time intensive, this may not always be feasible. We received funding from the American Recovery and Reinvestment Act to study the use and effectiveness of technology as a means to coach teachers. We compared face-to-face teacher coaching to Web-based coaching. The results suggest that Web-based coaching is an effective and promising approach for the use of technology to support and coach classroom teachers. The creation of a "coaching environment" facilitates instructional change through a coaching process. Our recent research results suggest that Web-based coaching is effective. Thus, the process of providing a supportive coaching environment may be more important than the physical location of the coaching activity because of these five critical functions of coaching:

1. To provide psychological support
2. To provide technical feedback
3. To analyze the appropriateness of the use and consequences of the target skills and application of skills
4. To adapt newly acquired skills to classroom students
5. To assist with sustained practice

It is argued that, through coaching, real, sustainable change based on reflective feedback and action can occur in the delivery of instructional methods and improvement in student performance.

Is Ongoing Coaching After the Initial COMPASS Consultation Really Necessary?

How necessary is it for consultants to follow up with teachers after the consultation is conducted? How many follow-up coaching sessions are necessary? How should the sessions be structured? Answers to these questions depend upon several factors:

- The purpose or outcome of the consultation
- The skills of the consultees (in this case, teachers)
- The attitude and motivation of the teacher
- The skills of the consultant
- The needs of the student

Very little research is available to guide consultants, teachers, and administrators with knowledge of what to expect for follow-up after consultation. What is very clear is that changes in teacher behavior and instruction using traditional professional development activities are limited (Guskey, 1986; Joyce & Showers, 2002).

An example of the necessity for follow-up comes from our own research and the research from others. We asked teachers to report how much training they received through traditional methods of professional development such as workshops, in-services, and conferences. We analyzed the number of training opportunities reported by teachers and whether teachers who had more training produced better quality IEPs for students with autism (Ruble, McGrew, Dalrymple, & Jung, 2010b). We were surprised to find no relationship between the two. In other words, both novice teachers as well as veteran teachers who had a lot of training had IEPs of similar quality, a finding that was unexpected because we thought that teachers who had more training about autism would produce IEPs more sensitive and specific to the needs of students with autism. There may be several reasons for these findings, including the increasing pressure teachers feel to align IEP objectives with state academic content standards. We found that many IEP goals came directly from state standards and were not modified for the individual student. But there are also other possible explanations.

Educational researchers Joyce and Showers (1983, 2002) examined the effectiveness of feedback, modeling, and didactic instruction in promoting active and sustainable change in teacher behavior and classroom instruction. The results provide striking evidence on what really works to create change. They examined types of in-service training of teachers by categories and rank-ordered the training categories according to their "level of impact" of the outcomes of the training event. The four levels of impact studied were the following:

1. Simple awareness of theory or practice
2. New understanding concerning the content and one's own knowledge related to the subject
3. Skill and proficiency with the materials
4. The transfer of new skills and understandings in the participant's own instructional setting

They found that only the last category of training, of which coaching is the primary example, was associated with any evidence of changes in teacher behavior and classroom instruction. Today, this remains the only professional development method that is associated with influencing student behavior, achievement, and success.

Although minimal results are produced from traditional training methods such as workshops, these methods of professional development may be useful to increase knowledge development of evidence-based practices in autism. It will be difficult to obtain sustainable change in teacher behavior if the outcome categories of 1, 2, and 3 are not achieved first. The resources provided in Chap. 3 and the information on evidence-based practices for students with autism are required knowledge of a COMPASS consultant (see Chap. 3, Table 3.2).

Performance Feedback

One method for assisting teachers in the implementation of knowledge gained from professional development activities is providing performance feedback. An example of a standard performance feedback procedure that is conducive to producing eventual change in teacher behavior involves meeting with the teacher to review the products of the intervention, such as a graph of student behavior, a list of the intervention implementation steps (Noell et al., 2005), a videotape review of the instructional situation, or examples of the student's work. Research on performance feedback shows that when teachers receive input on their performance, they are more likely to follow through with recommended teaching strategies (Jones, Wickstrom, & Friman, 1997; Martens, Hiralall, & Bradley, 1997; Noell et al., 2005). These findings suggest that the ways that follow-up occur and what happens during follow-up sessions may be important. We have implemented research-supported follow-up strategies in the COMPASS Coaching Protocol (Table 8.1).

Intervention Fidelity and Consultation Outcomes

In the COMPASS consultation framework, the concept of intervention fidelity is tied closely with the coaching process. Intervention fidelity refers to how well a teaching plan is implemented—a key ingredient in successful program implementation and achievement of positive student outcomes. In our own research, we found that the students who had teachers who were better able to follow through with teaching plans had better educational outcomes. We also learned that teachers needed several months following the initial consultation to implement the teaching plans with necessary fidelity. Recall that in our research, we conducted four follow-up teacher coaching sessions. In the series of follow-up sessions, the last and fourth coaching session—which represented the accumulation of overall implementation

Table 8.1 COMPASS Coaching Protocol

Step	Activity
1	Observe the student demonstrating each targeted skill/objective/goal. The observation might be from a video recording made prior to the coaching session
2	Review the Goal Attainment Scale (GAS) Form. For each objective, review and rate with the teacher the student's progress using the GAS Form from the observation, videotape of the observation, and/or data
3	Complete the Teacher Interview for Coaching Form for each objective. Discuss where and with whom the goal is taught and how the data are being kept. Discuss with the teacher aspects of the teaching plan that worked well during the observation and what missed opportunities or problems regarding the implementation of the teaching plan were observed. Evaluate together what changes might need to be made in the teaching plan and/or what details of the current plan need more attention
4	Complete summary activities. Within a week following the coaching session, a written summary of the coaching session using the COMPASS Coaching Summary Template will be mailed, faxed, or emailed to the teachers and parents/caregivers along with any enclosures agreed upon. Be sure that email addresses and phone numbers are correct. Set a date and time for next coaching session
5	Obtain completed evaluation and fidelity forms. Ask the teacher (and parent if present) to complete the COMPASS Coaching Feedback Form and the COMPASS Coaching Fidelity Checklist. The coach should also complete the fidelity checklist and other evaluation forms after each coaching session to monitor how well the procedures are implemented by the coach and the teacher

of the teaching plan—was the only session that was associated with student outcomes. In other words, it was not until well into the spring semester of the new calendar year that positive changes in teacher behavior were associated with positive student educational outcomes. These findings are based on our protocol of four coaching sessions spread across the school year every 4–6 weeks. The results may have been different if more sessions were conducted earlier in the year or on a more frequent basis.

What Skills Does a Coach Need?

Good coaches need more than the content knowledge acquired through most professional development activities. They also need to demonstrate the ability to apply knowledge and transfer their skills to others—that is, they need to possess the process skills necessary and effective for adult learning. Based on our experiences, in order to gain appropriate process skills, an effective coach will likely need direct teaching experiences that involve interacting and working with a number of students with ASD. ASD is one of the most heterogeneous disorders, and although all students with ASD share core features of social and communication impairments, they vary tremendously from one another. The self-evaluation tool in Chap. 3 can assist coaches in identifying areas for further training. Many coaches may not come from a teaching background. For these individuals, it is suggested that hands-on experiences be obtained through planned activities. These could include teaching in the classroom, working with a speech pathologist to teach functional communication, working with a school psychologist who teaches social skills, assisting an occupational therapist who works on motor and sensory issues, etc. The main point is to seek out a variety of experiences with a diverse array of children and professionals to increase direct experiences.

A good coach not only has skills to work well with students, but also has the ability to work well with adults; both of these are areas of skill development necessary for successful COMPASS consultation and coaching. To expect changes in teacher behavior, the coach must be able to successfully transfer knowledge and skill to the teacher. This transfer takes place within an ongoing and trusting relationship of coaching. The COMPASS Consultation Action Plan described in Chaps. 6 and 7 details a specific and systematic process that occurs prior to coaching. It sets the stage for collaboration and facilitates shared decision-making, prioritizing concerns, and solving problems.

Coaching, on the other hand, is the subsequent activity that helps put into practice the teaching plans developed during the consultation. It occurs with a focus on the context of the classroom and involves all aspects of knowledge and skill transfer that is bidirectional in its focus on plan implementation. The coaching and teacher are partners who are engaged in a shared activity with a common goal. In summary, consultation serves to set the goals and plan the strategies, and coaching helps put the plans into practice.

COMPASS Coaching Protocol

In the COMPASS model, after the initial consultation, the consultant conducts a minimum of four coaching sessions with the teacher throughout the year for optimal results.

The coaching protocol (outlined in Table 8.1) is used as a framework during each COMPASS coaching session. The protocol is composed of activities that serve as a guide for obtaining information on how well the teacher has followed through with teaching plans as well as for identifying current obstacles that require problem solving. Some obstacles may be obvious, while others may be more subtle and require follow-up questioning that goes beyond the standard protocol.

The standard COMPASS Coaching Protocol is made up of five steps. The first four steps involve the teacher and usually take about an hour and a half to complete. The final step occurs after the coaching session and is completed by the consultant/coach (we use these terms interchangeably).

The first coaching session may take longer than subsequent sessions to allow for time to further develop the teaching plans that were started during the consultation but not completed. The consultant also will need to explain and develop the

GAS Forms with the teacher and discuss how the progress data will be kept. A *Session 1 Coaching Protocol Form* is provided in the forms section.

The coach or teacher may also invite parents, therapists, assistants, or others who teach the student to the coaching sessions. However, with complicated schedules, their attendance may not be possible. Therefore, it may be necessary to discuss with the teacher methods of sharing the information. We recommend that the coach or the teacher videotape instruction periodically. This offers the teacher a good way to share teaching strategies and progress with others.

At the end of the chapter is a *COMPASS Coaching Checklist Form* that will help the coach organize the coaching materials. Also mentioned in the checklist are suggested books and resources. Information on the concept of structured teaching and activities based on the concept, information on the picture exchange communication system, information on teaching early social skills, and suggestions for dealing with behavior are helpful. In addition, the COMPASS information series of handouts are available online at http://www.ukautism.org/compass.php and can be printed off and shared with parents and teachers.

Step 1: Observe the Student

It is essential to observe the student performing each targeted objective during each coaching session. The most helpful observation is one that is done in person with the teacher and student. Classroom observation provides information that taping cannot. It helps the coach capture the student in the classroom with teaching assistants and classmates and provides a picture of the setup and overall interaction patterns. Sometimes, however, this requires changing the student's schedule, and changing the schedule may be disruptive for both the student and the teacher. Also, if the student is not at school, the observation cannot be done.

An alternative to live observation is the use of video recordings of the teacher–student instruction. We found that teachers have responded favorably to the use of a mini digital camcorder. Some comments made by teachers about the videotaping are provided in Fig. 8.1.

For teachers who prefer to tape the instruction prior to the coaching session, it is often helpful if they make the video as close in time to the coaching session as possible and on a day that the student is working optimally and can demonstrate his/her most consistent level of performance. Besides reducing disruptions, videotaping has other advantages as well. The video can be reviewed with other teachers and therapists and the student's parent(s). This permits other people to be involved and allows for immediate feedback and discussion. The video or observation does not have to be lengthy, but it does need to represent the targeted goal. The caveat of relying solely on taping for the review is that it minimizes the opportunities for live modeling and direct performance feedback. But taping also compensates for times when the student may be out of class due to sickness or may not be able to do the skill at

---

I am going to apply for a grant to get the mini camcorder for my classroom. It was extremely useful across many settings and very easy to use.

It was extremely useful to assist my student in meeting one of his goals. We videoed him then he would watch himself and tell us what he was doing wrong. He would want us to do it again so he could get it right.

I really loved the video camera. I have considered buying one for my family.

I developed a powerpoint with videos to share with teachers at new school [the] student will attend next year.

I have really enjoyed the coaching sessions. It has really helped to view videos together and discuss options and techniques.

The discussions and videos offered good insight on ways to help my student.

Watching the videos is a good way to observe and reflect on student progress!

Fig. 8.1 Comments from teachers about the use of videotaping

the usual level due to the change in schedule. There are benefits for both methods and also weaknesses. The best advice is to gauge the situation individually for each teacher and decide if the weaknesses outweigh the benefits for the observational approach used.

One last note is that although observation of the teacher demonstrating the instructional activity with the student is preferred, it is also helpful to have the person(s) who usually teaches the skill do the demonstration. We emphasize with teachers that the reason we like to observe them teaching a skill (in addition to the assistant) is that we assume that they will model the skill for the assistant and provide performance feedback to the assistant.

Step 2: Review the GAS Form

One of the goals of the first coaching session is to explain the *GAS Form* to the teacher. Ideally, it is suggested that the GAS Form be developed with the teacher. But due to time constraints, this might not be possible, and the consultant may have it ready for review with the teacher. The GAS Form will assist with progress monitoring for the remaining coaching sessions. We have provided a sample GAS Form (see Table 8.2), and a GAS Form template is located in the forms section of this chapter. Also, the case studies in Chap. 9 provide an example of how the GAS Form is used.

The GAS Form scale ranges from −2 (present levels of performance) to +2 (much more than expected level of outcome). Below are directions for creating a GAS Form for each one of the IEP objectives (for examples of completed GAS Forms, refer to the three case studies in Chap. 9).

Table 8.2 GAS Form

Rating	−2 Present level of performance	−1 Progress	0 Expected level of outcome (goal)	+1 Somewhat more than expected	+2 Much more than expected	Demonstrated for at least 2 weeks?
Skill observed? □ No □ Yes Goal changed? □ No □ Yes						

Creating a GAS Form

To begin writing the GAS Form, first start at the "0" level and write the measurable objective (we use goal and objective interchangeably) that is expected to be obtained by the end of the school year. Most skills are considered mastered if they can be independently demonstrated about 80% of the time. Then describe the student's present levels of performance at the −2 level. After completing these two activities, it will be easier to create benchmarks that describe progress (−1 level) from present levels (−2 level) to goal attainment (0). The additional two levels (+1 and +2) allow for progress above the expected level and provide opportunity to establish goals related to generalization.

The following information provides details for scaling the objectives across the five anchors (−2, −1, 0, +1, +2). Table 8.3 also illustrates how the various dimensions that can be used to determine skill progress are considered. The student can show progress if the skill is being performed at a higher frequency compared to the −2 level, or if there is less frequency of prompting or less restrictive forms of prompting. See Table 8.4 for examples of forms of prompts from least restrictive to most restrictive. The contexts within which the child can perform the skill and with whom they demonstrate the skill are also dimensions that can be considered for measuring progress.

Detailed instructions for completing each level are described.

0 Level: The objective (goal) as written in the IEP is at the Expected level of outcome, or 0 level. It is important to make sure that this objective is observable and measurable. How many times, over what period of time, and under what circumstance the behavior must occur is established. Chapter 5 provides additional guidance for writing high quality IEP objectives. Usually, the IEP has to be changed or updated after the consultation so that the goals generated from the consultation are accounted for in the IEP.

−2 Level: Once the goal is clearly established and agreed upon, the current level of performance is written as the −2 level. Sometimes, it is difficult to describe the student's present levels of performance because the IEP lacks behavioral descriptions. In this case, the information from the consultation, the latest assessment information, and teacher/parent observation can also be included in

Table 8.3 GAS: dimensions to consider for specifying progress

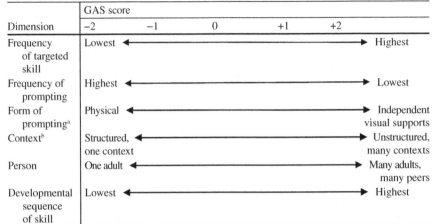

Dimension	GAS score				
	−2	−1	0	+1	+2
Frequency of targeted skill	Lowest ◄──────────────────► Highest				
Frequency of prompting	Highest ◄──────────────────► Lowest				
Form of prompting[a]	Physical ◄──────────────────► Independent visual supports				
Context[b]	Structured, one context ◄──────────────────► Unstructured, many contexts				
Person	One adult ◄──────────────────► Many adults, many peers				
Developmental sequence of skill	Lowest ◄──────────────────► Highest				

[a]See Table 8.4 for a description of hierarchy of prompts
[b]Context can refer to one-on-one, small group structured, small group unstructured, or unstructured or in any classroom instructional setting

the description. We are assuming that the student will not regress on this objective during the year and fall below the current level of performance. Based on our research of 79 children, none regressed below the −2 level over the school year. For example, Anthony's GAS Form (Chap. 9) has a description of his current performance related to the skill at the −2 level.

−1 Level: This level indicates what behaviors the student will demonstrate that represent progress toward the goal. We aim to make the skill at level −1 to be about 50% of the targeted goal in level 0. Also included is the frequency and type of prompting (e.g., verbal or physical cues). For example, if the student is expected to perform the skill four of five times independently (0 level) and is currently performing the skill two of five times (−2 level) with physical prompting, progress might be stated at four of five times with physical prompting (−1 level) or one of five times independently (−1 level). Both descriptions could be written because they both depict progress between levels −2 and 0. Other descriptors to measure accomplishment toward the IEP goal—such as number and type of cues (e.g., verbal, physical, gestural, or visual), number of tasks to complete, and environmental context or person(s) (e.g., teacher, other adults, peers, at recess, in the lunchroom, etc.)—are specified. Refer to Anthony's GAS Form (Chap. 9). Notice that the parenthetical information represents how performance may vary for that particular skill level. If performance is observed at the level denoted by at least one of the parenthetical descriptions, then the student is showing progress toward the goal. For Anthony progress beyond his present levels of performance would mean that when he is presented with a task, he will start and complete at least two tasks without any aggression. The criterion of two is about 50% of the targeted criterion of three (we rounded up 1.5–2 in this case).

Table 8.4 Examples of supports for enhancing independent skills following initial verbal direction: least restrictive to most restrictive prompts

Work behavior	Visual supports	Physical structure	Gestures	Verbal cues	Physical prompts
Remains seated	Provide work-reward schedule	Use corner seating	Point down	"Stay in your seat"	Place hands on child's shoulders
Remains in the group	Place child's photo on chair or book	Use furniture etc. to indicate boundaries of group area; Give the child a specific mat to sit on; position adult next to child	Point to area to go to	"Get back with the group"	Guide the child back to group by taking hand
Waits for instructions	Use "Wait" picture or gesture	Create distraction-free work area	Palm out	"Wait behind me"	Prompt the child to place hands on lap
Follows work-reward routine	Present 2-step visual schedule of work and reward	Create distraction-free work area	Point to first and then picture cue	"Time to work and get out your books"	Use hand over hand prompting
Initiates work activities	Use "Stop" and "Go" pictures	Set up designated work area; Set up materials so that starting point is clear	Point to picture schedule or activity	"Get out your paper and pencil and work"	Use hand over hand prompting for the first step of the task
Completes a sequence of tasks	Use visual schedule with pictures of work activities; have model of each sequence	Set up work shelf with different tasks labeled to correspond with visual schedule	Point to picture; sign	"Do the puzzle next?"	Prompt the child to raise hand to get assistance (e.g., touch child's elbow)
Asks for help when needed	Provide card illustrating what to do when the child needs help (e.g., raise hand)	Set up work situations in which the child will need help; Stand close by to respond promptly	Point to picture; sign	"Do you need help?"	Prompt the child to raise hand to get assistance (e.g., touch child's elbow)
Persists to completion	Provide pictures indicating the task steps	Choose tasks with clear end points; Present a limited number of materials	Point to visual cues of work routine	"Look, do your work"	Use hand over hand prompting as needed
Indicates when finished	Provide card illustrating what to do when finished (e.g., raise hand)	Provide a "finished box"	Point to finish picture or sign	"Put your paper in folder when done"	Prompt the child to raise hand or exchange picture indicating "finished"

+1 Level: This level indicates the student is making more progress than anticipated. The +1 level is represented by measurable progress that is about 50% greater than the skill description depicted at the 0 level. A score of +1 indicates that the student is able to perform the skill with more independence, or with more people, or in different settings and allows the generalization of the skill to be measured. Thus, the frequency of the skill is increased 50% above the stated objective or the skill is performed with less prompting, or more independently, or with peers, or in different contexts. See Anthony's GAS Form for an example. Note that if he made progress above the expected level and at the +1 level, he would need to be able to start and complete five tasks with no aggression. Five is about 50% more than three (again we rounded up 4.5–5 in this case).

+2 Level: This level indicates the student is performing significantly more than expected. For example, if Anthony was completing at least six independent work tasks with no aggression, he would achieve a +2 GAS score. The frequency of the skill may be 100% more than performed at the expected level of outcome. It also allows for further demonstration of generalization and independence. It may also represent the same function of the skill being performed using a different form or at a higher developmental level (e.g., the student uses a vocalization instead of a picture to make a request).

Setting the criteria for each level is important. As mentioned, the general rule is that level −1 should be reduced by about ½ or 50% of level 0 for frequency of performance and increased by about ½ for needed prompts for performance. In other words, the student is performing the skill about 50% less often and/or with about 50% more prompts. For example, a skill that is set to occur four of five times for level 0 would be reduced to two of five times at level 1; two verbal cues, might be increased to three to four verbal/gestural cues.

Following the same thought, level +1 would be incrementally scaled up by increasing performance by ½ of level 0 or by decreasing prompts by ½ of level 0. The scaling needs to be related to the skill as written in level 0 and make sense. It might not make sense to raise the level to four of five times since doing many skills at 80% is considered mastery (except in situations of safety and hygiene, etc.). But going from two verbal cues to one or going from working for 5 min to working for 8 would be appropriate. Level +2 would then increase by 100% or double what is written for level 0. This format helps keep the increments between the levels as even as possible. More examples of completed GAS Forms can be found in the case studies in Chap. 9.

Whatever criteria are set, they are carefully reviewed during the coaching session to ensure that they are truly measurable and observable and make sense. If in the first two coaching sessions they are found to need modification to make them clearer or more measurable, they are amended at that time with the teacher. This should be a document that helps the teacher and team members really use the IEP as a meaningful document for teaching and tracking progress. If something is not working, then the coaching sessions help problem-solve a solution. It is important to emphasize that data need to be collected by the teaching staff on each goal on a regular basis. The observation of student performance at coaching time is not for the sole basis of measuring progress but is also intended to create a good springboard for discussion.

At each remaining coaching session the GAS Form is reviewed as part of the COMPASS Coaching Protocol. The teacher's input and the observation are used to rate the GAS Form and a discussion about ways to keep data and whether the levels seen are accurate may take place. The consultant's observation rating is noted on the form as well. The teacher is reminded that her data and observation may be somewhat different than what was observed by the consultant, but that it is helpful to understand why there might be an inconsistency in ratings. If the skill was not observed, this is also indicated. Also noted on the form is any change to the goal since the last observation, and whether the student has been performing at the level for at least 2 weeks according to teacher report and data.

Step 3: Complete Teacher Interview for Coaching Form

The *Teacher Interview for Coaching Form* is completed during each coaching session with the teacher. It helps provide structure to the coaching session and a focus on conditions under which each objective is taught. Sometimes, the teacher says she just has not worked on this objective at all or sometimes that the assistant works on this so the teacher knows little about it. Talk about practical ways to fit teaching the objective into the teaching day or increase the frequency with which the skill is taught. If the objective is primarily targeted or practiced in other settings and with other people discuss ways to monitor and exchange ideas about consistency, progress, and assurance that the teaching plans are being implemented as written. Discuss other ways to possibly share with parents if they are not part of the coaching session for generalization.

The Teacher Interview for Coaching Form includes informal discussion regarding the details of the teaching plan for each objective. This helps the teacher express what concerns he may have or what may not be understood. It is helpful to discuss the teaching plan after observing each skill. This form allows the consultant to discuss possible adjustments to make with the plan and to seek input from the teacher regarding her own observations of what went well during the instructional demonstration or what missed opportunities were observed. The form will encourage discussion on why progress is being made or why progress is slow or not being made. Remember to consider the personal and environmental challenges and supports that are impacting skill development positively or negatively and discuss information using these terms. Sometimes, more environmental supports need to be in place, perhaps more visuals, for the student to be successful. Sometimes, the skill is not being taught or practiced enough. Sometimes, parents or school personnel may not know enough about the skill to help with generalization, or they may be doing something that is counter to learning. The teaching plan is viewed as a fluid document that is able to be adjusted in ways that maximize student engagement and progress over time. We suggest that the coach use technology, such as a laptop, for each coaching session to update the teaching plan so that the plan in place is the most current plan.

Sharing strategies and what is working is an important part of any plan. In everyday situations there are changes such as a new teaching assistant, a family moves, a baby is born into the family, or a child is sick that create or exacerbate personal or environmental challenges. These need to be noted and supports put in place when necessary. Document what additional environmental supports need to be put in place and what methods will be used to make this happen before the next coaching session. Sometimes, demonstrating the skill with a videotape of the skill being taught to another student is helpful for the teacher and the student. Using materials that the teacher has or materials the coach has brought as part of a demonstration also may be helpful. Figure 8.2 demonstrates a sample of a discussion during a coaching session regarding a social skill.

Step 4: Summary Activities

Review with the teacher the information that will be provided after the session using the *COMPASS* as a guide and sent to the teacher and parent (an example of a completed summary is provided in Chap. 9, the first case study Anthony). Especially review agreements on what will be the focus and emphasis for teaching each objective and any changes that have been made. Make sure that the teacher understands exactly how plans will be implemented and has committed to trying ideas that were agreed upon. If there is an assistant or others at the school who need the information and are not present, be sure there is a plan to translate the information to them and that there is a way to ensure consistency in implementation of the plans.

Make sure the participants know how to reach the coach by e-mail and how often they check their email. Phone numbers also can be exchanged so that last-minute changes can be conveyed. Set up the time for the next coaching session. Make a list of any materials that will be sent to the participants or brought to the next coaching.

A COMPASS Coaching Summary Template that will help format the summary of the session is included in the forms section of this chapter. This report should be completed as soon as possible and emailed or mailed to teacher and parents. It includes updates to the teaching plan so the plan is current. It may also be possible to use the form itself and write on it directly during the coaching session. A copy can be made and given to the teacher immediately. It will also be necessary to mail a copy to the caregiver if the caregiver is not present during the coaching session.

This excerpt is from the third coaching session. It begins after the teacher and consultant view a current video of the child demonstrating the skill with a new peer. They are playing a matching memory game.

C=Consultant; T=Teacher

C:Is the peer new?
T: She's a student we've had all year, but she was absent during a couple of the other tapings. She's a very good partner; however, you can see she'll kind of take over and just plow right along and take all those cues. But she is one that we like to pair her with.
C: Uh huh. Yeah. And she's very good.
T: Right.
C: ...at giving the cues. And is a good peer. Okay so, what do you think worked well or could have worked better when you watched the video?
T: I think the symbol and having the cue cards worked very well. Also, having an activity that's of interest to the child. She really likes Dora, so that's a game that will keep her attention through enough exchanges. I guess not that it's not working, but I'm still curious how to get her a little more engaged during the game. You can tell you know, she is not responding or really paying a lot of attention to the peer that she is playing with. You know, I feel like we're coaching her saying, "Look at her." "Tell her this..." and you know, "Stop," "Let's say good game at the end." and you know you could tell as soon as she was done she was ready to leave.
C: Was that the first time they played that game?
T: No. They probably played that one at that point two or three times...so we've worked on that one a few times. That game. Probably not the same card matches, but that game...the memory format.
C: Let's look at the GAS form.
T: Okay.
T: Umm, I get stuck with the amount of prompting we're allowed to do and include it. 'Cause she will keep performing at the -1level (which allows for prompting) and play through four exchanges, but she will not do that independently. If we were to say play together and get the two of them started and then leave. She would probably walk off too.
C: One thing we need to do is look at the coaching summary from last session because we had a similar situation we brought up last time that we talked about, but we'll wait for that in a second when we get to the teaching plan to discuss some specific ideas. I think with a peer like this who is very directive, you have lots of opportunities. The peer can take over the directiveness without the adult doing it. And right now, they both are really focused on the adult.
T: Right. And we have put into the instruction that card where they flip the card more often to indicate "my turn." And I think the more they do that together, that's going to become a little pattern.
C: Yes. So it's like the other ones. I see what you're saying, like where to rate her given the adult prompting. Looking at where she started off at -2, she really wasn't doing any real turn-taking. Although she did have an idea of what go play and kind of generally what that meant, she had no idea of what to do with a peer. Clearly she is not at that level anymore. And last time I think we rated her, let's see...a -1.5. So, let's see the way that we have this for -1...She's also doing it through multiple exchanges. She did stay there for more than, at least four exchanges And..so the question again is the prompting. So I wonder what would

Fig. 8.2 Example of a discussion during a coaching session.

C=Consultant; T=Teacher

happen what again if the adult wasn't there and the peer was there. You had the nice visuals. You've got the routine set. If they could go through a couple of exchanges together...

T: Right. I will try that tomorrow because often I will put them down to do things, you know kind of down on the floor with the big group. But if I would try those two again with that activity. I would be curious also to see if the peer can keep it going.

C: Yeah. You know what, why don't you try that, then let me know. Shoot me an email, or maybe I can get the video. Because I'm just real curious too.

T: Okay. Yeah, I can try that. I might be able to get that today.

C: Yeah, because I can see some real progress she's made. So let's look at the teaching plan. You've got a sociable peer. And setting up the situations of interest, which has been a challenge, but you've found some of those that are working.

T: Right.

C: Direct instruction...and you've got the card there and have you used a social story? Or any role playing?

T: Yes. We've used a social story, and I also put a social story on my iPad about taking turns. And we've been talking a lot about taking turns and kind of modeling it. You know two teachers would model it for her and how to take turns.

C: Okay you've got all these things in place. Here are a couple ideas for that.

T: Okay.

C: Set the children so that they are across from each other.

T: Okay.

C: If you've got a narrow enough table so they could be exchanging that back and forth, that will make it easier for them to exchange the materials. Also, Right now the two children are centered on looking at that adult.

T: Okay.

C: So if the children could be moved so that they are facing each other...

T: Okay, that's a very good idea. I think sometimes I set things up for filming that way, but that's a very good idea. So they can have each other directly across from one another.

C: Yes, and then let them know that they know how to play the game, and they're going to play the game themselves. You may need to give some extra directions ahead of time, a little bit extra cuing to the peer, but she seems like kind of a natural for doing that.

T: Yes I thought about doing that. The other day she helped and was said she was going to like this.

C: The way that we wrote this goal means that you can give the peer as many cues as you want. We really wrote this for the peer to be cuing her, so that it will generalize more when the children are playing with each other and an adult isn't around. If the peer doesn't move the game along, you can cue the peer. And I will think they will be able to do this through four exchanges.

T: Okay.

C: And I think it says, "how many?" Three different activities, so once they get it, I don't think that's going to be a problem.

T: And we have an expression game and a ball game. So we have been trying to do it across different activities.

C: How many times a day is that worked on?

T: Mmm. Probably two, sometimes just one depending on our schedule.

Fig. 8.2 (continued)

C=Consultant; T=Teacher
C: And you're keeping data on that?
T: Yes. Twice a week.
C: And then you and the assistant are working on that. Anyone else?
T: Yes, I'm working on that, and the teaching assistant. And then I have two high schoolers who have been coming in. So I'm trying to teach them how to work on that also so that she has as many opportunities as possible.
C: Okay. That's great.
C: Okay. Do you have other questions?
T: No, but these are some good things that I will work on. Probably my only questions are on data keeping. I'm keeping the data you know. Also, she has an older brother who is in high school, and he is coming to do an observation for the week next week. So I might be curious to see how he feels she's doing on these goals.
C: That will be interesting.
T: Yes.
C: Yes. And it will be a nice carryover at home. Okay, what we've got is the next session for March 23rd. and we have it at the same time.
T: Okay. Can we try to make it any later that day?
(the conversation continues a few minutes about scheduling the next coaching session; discussion of getting videos, etc)
C: Any other questions you have?
T: No. That's all. Thank you.

Fig. 8.2 (continued)

Step 5: Fidelity Forms and Evaluation

Before starting the coaching session, review the forms section for the *COMPASS Coaching Feedback Form* and the *COMPASS Coaching Fidelity Checklist.* These are both designed for the teacher to complete. But the fidelity checklist can also be used by the coach to ensure that all steps of the coaching protocol are followed. These forms provide information to better understand how the teacher is feeling about the coaching session (satisfaction) and what might need to be adjusted prior to the next coaching session (fidelity). We suggest that the fidelity forms be used every other session to ensure that the steps of the coaching session are being implemented as designed. The satisfaction form is distributed at the end of coaching, but can also be used as a means to evaluate the process of the coaching sessions and used every other session as well.

Included in the forms section are two additional forms that evaluate the quality of both the student's engagement during instruction (*Autism Engagement Rating Scale*) and the teacher's characteristics of instruction (*Teacher Engagement Rating Scale*). These forms are helpful with identifying aspects of the teacher instruction to consider during coaching sessions. Engagement is a term often used in autism research as a critical variable in effective treatment programs. Research studies on intervention suggest that children should be meaningfully engaged at least 25 h a week (National Research Council, 2001). The term—engagement, however, has not been used consistently and can be vague. Thus, our rating scale on child engagement was created to help define what we mean by engagement and what we think would be helpful for teachers to understand when they are trying to increase the meaningful engagement of their students with autism. We found that when compared to students who had

Down syndrome and similar cognitive and language skills to the students with autism, students with Down syndrome (DS) were more "in sync" with the classroom activities (Ruble & Robson, 2007). They showed more consistency or congruency between the topic being discussed and their responsiveness to the instruction. Students with autism, on the other hand, were more compliant compared to their counterparts with DS. That is, the students with autism "looked" engaged because they were with the group, sitting at their desk, working with the appropriate tools, etc. But on closer inspection, they were less likely to be working on the same materials or be on the same topic. We refer to this as "consistency" or how closely the teacher's goal directed behavior for the child is aligned with the child's own goal directed behavior. We used this form and the teacher engagement form to evaluate whether teacher and student engagement changes over time as a result of the coaching sessions.

We found that the coaching sessions did indeed help those teachers who were rated lower in engagement at the beginning of the year and improved their engagement at the end of the year (Ruble, McGrew, & Toland, 2010). Teachers who were rated high on engagement at the beginning of the year, stayed high on engagement throughout the coaching sessions. The items on the teacher engagement form come from research on student development. We examined these features of adult–student interaction and reported findings in a study with parents (Ruble, McDuffie, & King, 2009). We found that children of parents who were more responsive and less directive had better social initiation skills based on parent report. Research is currently being conducted to see if the same happens for teachers. It is common to find teachers of students with autism using a directive interaction style during instruction. Often, a teacher uses verbal or physical cues and prompts repeatedly. For these teachers, it is important to help them become aware of their style and the potential missed opportunities for effective instruction that encourages initiation, independence, and problem solving in the student. If a student is being directed constantly and not given ample time to respond or learn to initiate a skill independently, then difficulties initiating skills, problem solving, learning to use trial and error, developing independence, and generalizing skills can result.

Terminating the Consultation

The consultant and the teacher may agree that coaching will continue until the student has reached a certain level or when the teacher feels the teaching plan is fully implemented and the student is making progress. We found that it is optimal to consult with the teacher throughout the school year because it took at least three sessions to see significant progress toward implementing the teaching plans with good fidelity. It is helpful to have this agreement in place before the consultation begins. Too often, consultants and coaches are called in when there is a crisis, and when the immediate crisis is over the consultant leaves. Although there may be a crisis that initiated the consultation process or one that occurs along the way, the consultant role is quite different in COMPASS. Unfortunately, families move, teachers change, and other unforeseen events happen. It is hoped the information and activities that have been put together for each student will follow the student.

Appendix A   Instructions for Completing Chapter 8 Forms

1. Review all forms prior to conducting a coaching session. The *Session 1 Coaching Protocol* is adapted for the first session. The *Standard COMPASS Coaching Protocol* describes the steps to complete for the remaining coaching sessions.
2. The *Coaching Checklist* provides a list of forms, information, and equipment to gather and use for the coaching session. Attached at the bottom of the checklist is information on the date and time of the next coaching session that can be torn from the bottom and given to the teacher.
3. The *Goal Attainment Scale (GAS) Form* is used to monitor the progress of the measurable objective. Indicate the student's rating following each observation during the coaching session. Also indicate if the skill was actually observed or not and if the goal changed since the last session. Note the domain of the skill and whether the student has been performing at the level observed for at least 2 weeks.
4. The *Teacher Interview for Coaching Form* provides the questions to ask during the coaching session. It is recommended that the teacher be provided a copy of this interview at the time that the questions are presented. This assists the teacher in organizing information in advance.
5. The *COMPASS Coaching Summary Template* provides a recommended outline for the coaching summary report. What was observed is described first, followed by the discussion for each objective. The discussion information comes from the responses to the *Teacher Interview for Coaching Form*. Goal attainment for each of the three objectives is reported. What is observed and what the teacher reports as the level of skill most consistently performed are noted. Finally, the last part of the coaching summary is a specific description of future plans. Future plans include the date and time of the next coaching session. It also includes any descriptions of modifications and/or adaptations to make in the teaching plan or instructional approach. Other information and resources might also be included. An example of a completed summary is in the case study of Anthony.
6. The next two forms are designed to evaluate the teacher perceptions of the coaching session. The *COMPASS Coaching Feedback Form* assesses satisfaction and the *COMPASS Coaching Fidelity Checklist* assesses the degree to which the consultant followed and adhered to the procedures of the coaching session. It is suggested that these forms be given every other session so that the teacher does not grow fatigued with completing many forms. The forms can be administered together or separately, every other time. The coach reviews the forms and makes adjustments based on the feedback.
7. After each coaching session, the *COMPASS Coaching Impressions Scale* is completed by the consultant. Note that item 10 is the most important question and refers to how well the teacher followed through with the recommendations and teaching plan.
8. Two additional measures—the *Autism Engagement Rating Scale* and the *Teacher Engagement Rating Scale*—provide information on the quality of the student's engagement and teacher instruction during the teaching situations. Higher scores

reflect higher quality engagement. Definitions for each of the items are provided. This information informs the consultant about areas of skills to target with the teacher on the quality of the student and teacher engagement.

9. Two types of data collection examples are provided. It is important to encourage teachers to feel comfortable creating their own or adapting the current forms that best suit their needs and circumstances. Examples of completed data sheets are provided in case study 1—Anthony.

Appendix B   Session 1 Coaching Protocol

With teacher/parent/others:

1. Check to see that the teacher received the *Consultation Summary Report.*
2. Complete teaching plans for any objectives that were not finished at the consultation and review and edit any plans that now need to be changed.
3. Explain the purpose and review the draft *GAS Form* that is completed with the teacher or was completed prior to the coaching session. Make any changes based on teacher input and be sure to word each skill so that it is measurable and observable and that everyone agrees to the meaning.
4. Then proceed with Steps 2–7 of the standard protocol that will be used for the follow-up coaching sessions.

Note: The objective may not have been worked on at all or very little prior to Coaching Session 1, but it is still important to observe the student performing the skill as a base for discussion and for rating of the GAS Form.

Appendix C   Standard COMPASS Coaching Protocol

1. Check that the teacher and parent received information from the prior coaching and that it is available and was understood. Also determine if changes have occurred, including any changes to the IEP, since the summary was sent.
2. Review the *COMPASS Coaching Fidelity Checklist* before the session and make sure that each component is followed (the teacher will complete the fidelity checklist following the consultation).
3. For each skill/objective/goal, the following steps are followed in order. Repeat for each.

   (a) Observe the student performing the skill either live or from video recording.
   (b) Review and rate the *GAS Form* for that skill, also obtain teacher's assessment of the student's most consistent level of progress based on data.
   (c) Complete the *Teacher Interview for Coaching Form* on that skill.
   (d) Review the teaching plan (see Chap. 7) that was generated from the COMPASS consultation for this skill and make changes as discussion warrants.
   (e) Problem-solve any additional personal and environmental challenges and supports that may need to be addressed, modified, added, or maintained (provide other assistance such as use of demonstration, role plays, or modeling the instruction, and making materials).
   (f) Gather sample data forms from the teacher.

4. Inform the teacher that a summary of this coaching session and an updated *Teaching Plan* (if applicable) and an updated *GAS Form* (if applicable) will follow shortly. Decide if any additional information might be useful and either send it or provide a reference for it. Examples of helpful information are the Web sites described in Chap. 3 and the *Evidence-based Resources for Teachers Checklist* in the forms section of Chap. 7.
5. Set date and time for next coaching and make sure that email and phone numbers for questions are easily accessible for the teacher.
6. Ask the teacher to complete the *COMPASS Coaching Fidelity Checklist* and the *COMPASS Consultation Satisfaction Questionnaire*. To avoid burdening the teacher with paperwork, these forms can be given after every other session. They can also be mailed or faxed to the consultant after completion.
7. After coaching, complete the following forms. These forms are optional, but they are also designed to help the consultant assess and recognize possible areas to target for the next session.
   • Autism Engagement Rating Scale
   • Teacher Engagement Rating Scale
   • Coaching Impressions Scale
8. Write the summary and update the *Teaching Plan* and *GAS Form* if needed and send via email to teacher and regular mail to parents and teacher. Enclose any promised information.

Appendix D   COMPASS Coaching Checklist

Student's Name:_____ Coaching Date:_____

Coach's Packet (Standard Forms)	Equipment*
□ Coaching Protocol □ Teacher Interview for Coaching Form □ Blank GAS Forms (+1 extra for teacher) □ Blank Teaching Plan □ COMPASS Coaching Summary Template □ Enclosures not mailed with report □ Resources for Teachers Checklist (Chap. 7) □ Autism Engagement Rating Scale □ Teacher Engagement Rating Scale □ COMPASS Coaching Fidelity Checklist □ COMPASS Coaching Feedback Form □ Multiple Trials Data Sheet □ Activity-based Data Sheet	□ 2 tape recorders □ 2 audio tapes for coaching □ 1 audio tape for dictation □ Extra batteries □ Laptop □ Video camera/tapes □ Tripod □ Extension cord

Additional Information	Coach's Forms (Child Specific)
□ Contact Information □ Directions □ Schedule/Calendar	□ COMPASS consultation report and/or coaching summary report □ IEP □ GAS Form □ Teaching Plans

*This equipment is optional and depends on the information the coach wants to collect.

Other resources and print materials: _____

Teacher: _____ School: _____

Next Coaching Session Date and Time: _____

Notes: _____

_____cut_____

Teacher:

Your next coaching session will be _____ from_____ a.m./p.m. to _____a.m./p.m.

If you have any questions and/or concerns, please feel free to contact me at:

_____

Goal Attainment Scale (GAS) Form

Student's Name:_____   Observer:_____   Date:_____   Coaching I II III IV

Instructions: Indicate rating, if skill was directly observed, and whether the goal has changed since the last observation.

Skill Level	-2 Present level of performance	-1 Progress	0 Expected level of outcome (GOAL)	+1 Somewhat more than expected	+2 Much more than expected	Domain of Goal*	Demo for at least 2 weeks?**
1. Rating:_____ Was skill observed? ☐ no ☐ yes Has goal changed? ☐ no ☐ yes							
2. Rating:_____ Was skill observed? ☐ no ☐ yes Has goal changed? ☐ no ☐ yes							
3. Rating:_____ Was skill observed? ☐ no ☐ yes Has goal changed? ☐ no ☐ yes							

* Note: "Domain" refers to social, communication, learning skill, adaptive behavior, motor/sensory or academic goals.
**Has student been able to perform at criterion level for at least two weeks?

Appendix E   Teacher Interview for Coaching Form

Date: _____ Teacher's Name: _____

Interviewer: _____ Coaching Session Number: I, II, III, IV

Instructions: For each goal, answer the following questions using the GAS Form.

GAS Objective # 1

1. Skill domain—*circle the domain:*
   0 = Academic   1 = Social   2 = Communication   3 = Learning/Work Skills
   4 = Motor/Sensory   5 = Self-help   6 = Behavior
2. How many times a day/week is this skill worked on? _____ day/week (specify)
3. Do you keep data on the skill? □ Yes (if so, please provide an example)
   □ No (if not, provide examples to teacher)
4. What teaching methods are used to teach the skill?
5. Who usually instructs the skill? *Circle all that apply.*
   1 = teacher 2 = assistant 3 = speech language pathologist 4 = peers 5 = other
6. Did the coach provide modeling/demonstration of skill? □ Yes □ No

GAS Objective # 2

1. Skill domain—*circle the domain:*
   0 = Academic   1 = Social   2 = Communication   3 = Learning/Work Skills
   4 = Motor/Sensory   5 = Self-help   6 = Behavior
2. How many times a day/week is this skill worked on? _____
   day/week (specify)
3. Do you keep data on the skill? □ Yes (if so, please provide an example) □ No
   (if not, provide examples to teacher)
4. What teaching methods are used to teach the skill?
5. Who usually instructs the skill? *Circle all that apply.*
   1 = teacher 2 = assistant 3 = speech language pathologist 4 = peers 5 = other
6. Did the coach provide modeling/demonstration of skill? □ Yes □ No

GAS Objective # 3

1. Skill domain—*circle the domain:*
   0 = Academic   1 = Social   2 = Communication   3 = Learning/Work Skills
   4 = Motor/Sensory   5 = Self-help   6 = Behavior
2. How many times a day/week is this skill worked on? _____ day/week
   (specify)
3. Do you keep data on the skill? □ Yes (if so, please provide an example) □ No
   (if not, provide examples to the teacher)
4. What teaching methods are used to teach the skill?
5. Who usually instructs the skill? *Circle all that apply.*
   1 = teacher 2 = assistant 3 = speech language pathologist 4 = peers 5 = other
6. Did the coach provide modeling/demonstration of skill? □ Yes □ No

Appendix F   COMPASS Coaching Feedback Form

Name (optional):_____ Date:_____

Please rate each question 1 (not very much) through 4 (very much). Use "NA" if "not applicable."

A. How much did the coaching session:

		Not very much			Very much	
1.	Support you to help the child reach his/her IEP objectives	1	2	3	4	NA
2.	Support you to implement strategies to reach the three targeted objectives	1	2	3	4	NA
3.	Support you to try new interventions	1	2	3	4	NA
4.	Cause you stress	1	2	3	4	NA

B. How helpful were components of the coaching session:

		Not very much			Very much	
5.	Discussions	1	2	3	4	NA
6.	DVDs/video recordings	1	2	3	4	NA
7.	Goal Attainment Scale (GAS) Form	1	2	3	4	NA

C. How much did you feel that the coach was:

		Not very much			Very much	
8.	A good listener	1	2	3	4	NA
9.	Nonjudgmental	1	2	3	4	NA
10.	Able to offer ideas and strategies	1	2	3	4	NA
11.	Encouraging	1	2	3	4	NA

D. Please add other comments (and use the back if necessary):

Appendix G   COMPASS Coaching Fidelity Checklist

Teacher's Name_____ Date_____

1. We reviewed the consultation/coaching written summary report and answered questions.	NO	YES
2. We reviewed the most current teaching plan and updated the written plan to reflect current teaching strategies for each objective.	NO	YES
3. We evaluated the goal attainment of the child's most current level of progress on the three skills.	NO	YES
4. After the observation of each skill, the consultant began the discussion by asking the teacher about thoughts of what was observed.	NO	YES
5. We discussed at least one idea (what teaching methods to keep in place or what teaching methods to consider changing) for each objective.	NO	YES
6. If the student was not making as much progress as desired on an objective, we discussed the student's personal challenges that might be impacting progress on skills.	NO	YES
7. If the student was not making as much progress as desired on an objective, we also discussed the student's environmental challenges that might be impacting progress on skills.	NO	YES
8. To counter the personal challenges related to an objective, we identified at least one personal support (e.g., a reinforcer, strength) to continue to use, add, or adapt in the teaching plan.	NO	YES
9. To counter environmental challenges related to an objective, we identified at least one environmental support (e.g., instructional method, visual support) to continue to use, add, or adapt in the teaching plan.	NO	YES
10. We discussed other environmental factors (student, teacher, or caregiver related) that might be helping or hindering the student progress either directly (health issues) or indirectly (home or classroom issues) on accomplishment of the objective.	NO	YES
11. We reviewed and rated the GAS Form for each objective the teacher/student demonstrated.	NO	YES
12. We obtained the rating of the student's most consistent and representative level of progress over the past two-week period.	NO	YES
13. For each objective, we discussed how often the skill is taught, if data are being kept, and problem solved any data collection issues.	NO	YES
14. We discussed generalization plans (e.g., who else is working on this skill with the student; where else does the student practice this skill; how is information being shared with other school personnel about this skill) for each objective.	NO	YES
15. The overall tone set by the consultant during the session was collaborative? (e.g., positive tone; positive feedback: "I think you're doing a good job in the classroom"; providing information; elaboration; initiating joint activities: "Let's focus on social problems right now").	NO	YES
16. The overall tone set by the consultant during the session was empowering? (e.g., the consultant asked open-ended questions to encourage teacher problem solving and self-reflection; the consultant helped to develop teacher confidence in ability to impact change).	NO	YES

Appendix H   COMPASS Coaching Summary Template

Coaching Session   I   II   III   IV

Student: _____ Date: _____ School: _____

Teacher: _____ Consultant: _____

Others Present: _____

Communication Skill:

Observation:

Discussion:

Goal Attainment:

Social Skill:

Observation:

Discussion:

Goal Attainment:

Learning Skill:

Observation:

Discussion:

Goal Attainment:

Future Plans:

Appendix I   COMPASS Coaching Impressions Scale

Child's Name: _____ Date:_____

Coach's Name:_____

Coaching Session *(circle one)*: I II III IV

Teacher—Special Education

		Not very much				Very much
1.	Welcoming and ready	1	2	3	4	5
2.	Organized	1	2	3	4	5
3.	Frustrated	1	2	3	4	5
4.	Positive about progress	1	2	3	4	5
5.	Defensive	1	2	3	4	5
6.	Positive about child	1	2	3	4	5
7.	Expression of stress/anxiety	1	2	3	4	5

General Atmosphere at Coaching Session

		Not very much				Very much
8.	Observation related to goals*	1	2	3	4	5
9.	The teacher read the report/coaching summary	1	2	3	4	5
10.	The teacher has followed through with recommendations**	1	2	3	4	5

*This item refers to how well the skill that was demonstrated for rating represented the skill described on the Goal Attainment Scale Form.
**For item 10, if the teacher has implemented none of the components of the teaching plan, score "1"; if about 25% of the components were implemented, score "2"; if about 50% of components were implemented, score "3"; if about 75% of components were implemented, score "4"; if about 100% of components were implemented, score "5."

Appendix J Autism Engagement Rating Scale (Classroom Version)

Child's Name:_____ Activity: _____

Observation Date:_____ Observer:_____

Description of Session (circle): Baseline Coaching I, II, III, IV, Final Evaluation

Type of Instruction (circle): Large Group Small Group 1:1 Adult Independent

	Cooperation
1	*Refuses* to participate in activity.
1.5	*Limited* participation in activity.
2	*Partially* participates in activity.
2.5	*Frequently* participates in activity.
3	*Fully* participates in activity; may show enthusiasm for completing activity.

Observations/comments:

	Functionality
1	*Does not* use objects appropriately.
1.5	*Limited* appropriate use of objects.
2	Demonstrates *some* appropriate use of objects.
2.5	*Frequently* uses objects appropriately.
3	Is successful in *consistently* using objects appropriately. The child does not demonstrate inappropriate use of objects.

Observations/comments:

	Productivity
1	*Does not* lead to the targeted outcome. Play/task is *not* purposeful.
1.5	*Limited* progress is made toward targeted outcome. Purpose of play/task is *limited*.
2	*Some* progress is made toward targeted outcome. Play/task is *somewhat* purposeful.
2.5	*Significant* progress is made toward targeted outcome. Play/task is *generally* purposeful.
3	Targeted outcome is achieved. Play/task is *completely* purposeful.

Observations/comments:

	Independence
1	*Does not* complete task independently and requires *constant* physical prompts throughout activity and never responds
1.5	Requires *several* prompts to complete tasks. The child *rarely* responds to verbal or gestural prompts throughout activity.
2	May require *some* prompts to complete tasks. The child responds to verbal or gestural prompts *throughout* activity.
2.5	The child requires *minimal* verbal or gestural prompts *throughout* activity.
3	*Does not* require verbal or gestural prompts to complete tasks. The child completes tasks independently *throughout* activity.

Observations/comments:

	Consistency
1	Child's goal directed behavior is *completely* different from the teacher's goal directed behavior for the child.
1.5	Child's goal directed behavior is *mostly* different from the teacher's goal directed behavior for the child.
2	Child's goal directed behavior is *somewhat* consistent with the teacher's goal directed behavior for the child.
2.5	Child's goal directed behavior is *mostly* consistent with the teacher's goal directed behavior for the child.
3	Child's goal directed behavior is the *same* as the teacher's goal directed behavior for the child.

Observations/comments:

	Attention
1	Is *not* attentive during the entire activity. The child shows no interest in activity.
1.5	*Limited* attention to activities is shown. Interest is also *limited*.
2	Shows *some* attention to and interest in activity.
2.5	Is *frequently* attentive to activity.
3	Is *fully* attentive during entire activity.

Observations/comments:

Autism Engagement Rating Scale: Hints for Coding (Ruble et al., revised 2005)

Cooperation: Measures child's ability to cooperate with and participate in designated activity/play.

1   The child pulls away from teacher/parent and/or falls to the ground and refuses participation in an activity. The child may cry and/or tantrum. The child may also appear apathetic or unresponsive to attempts to engage him/her in an activity.

1.5   The child's behavior is consistent with the description above, but the child shows limited cooperation and participation. Tantrums may be less severe; however, the child may whine or show dislike before or during cooperating with or participating in an activity.

2   The child's overall behavior consists of both resistance to and cooperation with activities. The child may show dislike for the activity, but may still participate. The child does not actively refuse activity.

2.5   The child frequently participates in and cooperates with activities. The child may show dislike for an activity and initially resist, but the child does eventually participate in that activity. Minimal refusal to participate is shown.

3   During the entire session, the child consistently cooperates with and participates in all activities without resistance.

Functionality: Measures child's ability to use objects in their intended manner.

1   The child does not use objects in the manner in which they were designed to be used. Use of objects is completely nonfunctional (e.g., child taps pencil on forehead, mouths toy, etc.).

1.5   The child's appropriate use of objects is limited. The child may occasionally demonstrate correct use, such as briefly rolling a ball after mouthing it.

2   The child demonstrates both appropriate and inappropriate use of objects during the session. The child increasingly uses objects correctly.

2.5   The child frequently uses objects the way they were intended with occasional misuse of objects being demonstrated. On the whole, object use is appropriate and functional.

3   Objects are consistently used in the manner in which they were intended. Inappropriate use of objects is absent.

Productivity: Measures child's ability to engage in meaningful work or play behavior.

1   Play/task does not have a purpose and is not useful. The child does not work toward completing the designated task.

1.5   The child makes some limited effort toward task completion. Some behaviors are useful and aid the child in completing the task/playing, although the majority of behaviors are not relevant to the task.

2   The child makes some progress toward task completion. Play/task behaviors are somewhat useful and or purposeful.

2.5   The child's behavior is mostly goal-oriented and purposeful. Significant progress is made toward task completion.

3   All behavior is productive and oriented toward task completion. Task completion/play may lead to development of higher-level skills.

Independence: Measures child's ability to follow instructions and work on tasks without prompts.

1   The child requires constant physical assistance to complete tasks, such as hand-over-hand assistance. The child may also require physical guidance during periods of transition to new activities.

1.5   Many physical prompts are needed to complete task. Although verbal/gestural prompts may be given, the child rarely responds to these prompts and they do not assist with task completion.

2   Physical prompts are not needed for task completion. Verbal/Gestural prompts are successful in helping the child focus work independently.

2.5   Very few verbal/gestural prompts are required to assist the child in working independently.

3   The child can complete tasks without assistance and/or reminders after initial instruction.

Consistency: Measures how closely the teacher's goal directed behavior for the child is aligned with the child' goal directed behavior.

1   The teacher's goals for the child are inconsistent with the child's goal directed behavior. As an example, the child may be completing a puzzle about the alphabet while the teacher is instructing in science; the child may be putting toys in his mouth while the teacher is trying to get the child to play with toys functionally. The child's own goals are inconsistent with the teacher's goals for the child.

1.5   The teacher's goals for the child are largely inconsistent with the child's goals.

2   The teacher's goals for the child are somewhat consistent with the child's goal directed behavior. The child may be working on alphabet puzzle while the teacher is instructing the class in reading.

2.5   The child's and the teacher's goals are mostly the same.

3   The child and the teacher have the same goal directed behaviors, working with consistency on the same lesson. The child's work may be adapted, but the content is the same. As an example, the child may complete a puzzle about the letter "L" while the teacher instructs the class to color a sheet on the letter "L."

Attention: Measures the child's interest in and attention to an activity.

1   The child appears extremely disinterested in an activity. The child may refuse to look at task and engage in activity. The child may turn away from or ignore activity.

1.5   The child occasionally shows some interest in activity. The child may briefly glance at activity before redirecting attention.

2   The child both ignores and attends to activity. Task holds child's attention briefly.

2.5   The child is very attentive to task. Few periods of distraction/inattention are observed.

3   The child demonstrates sustained attention on task and is interested in task.

Appendix K Teacher Engagement Rating Scale
(Ruble et al., revised 2005)

Student:_____ Teacher _____

Date:_____ Observer:_____

Instruction (circle): Large Group   Small Group   1:1 Adult   Independent

Description of Session (circle): Baseline Coaching I, II, III, IV, Final Evaluation

	Maintenance of Interaction		Directiveness
1	*Does not* attempt to help the student to be productive in student's interactions with objects and does not demonstrate or facilitate an object's proper use.	1	*Repeatedly and intensely* attempts to direct the student's immediate attention and/or behavior.
1.5	Makes *limited* attempt to foster productivity in interactions with objects and makes minimal effort to demonstrate or facilitate an object's proper use.	1.5	*Frequently* attempts to direct the student's immediate attention and/or behavior.
		2	Makes *some* attempts to direct the student's attention and/or behavior.
2	Makes *some* attempts to maintain productivity, to demonstrate an object's proper use, or to help the student use an object appropriately.	2.5	Maintains student's interest by directing the student's attention and/or behavior on a *limited* basis.
2.5	Makes *frequent* attempts to and is successful in maintaining productivity. The teacher demonstrates and facilitates an object's proper use.	3	Tailors directiveness based on the student's behavior *throughout* by allowing adequate response time and/or independence.
3	Is successful in helping the student to be productive in interactions with objects and/or others *throughout* the session using a wide variety of different approaches.		

	Initiation		Level of Movement/Participation
1	Is *apathetic and does not* attempt to direct the child's attention and/or behavior.	1	*Does not* move with the child and his/her activities and does not participate with the child.
1.5	Is passive but makes *limited* attempt to initiate with the child.	1.5	Makes *limited* movements with the child and makes few attempts to participate with the child.
2	Initiates *some* of the time with the child.	2	*Somewhat* moves with the child and participates some of the time.
2.5	Initiates positively with the child *frequently.*		
3	Initiates positively with the child *throughout.*	2.5	*Frequently* moves with the child and *frequently* participates with the child.
		3	Moves with the child and his/her activities and encourages participation *throughout.*

	Level of Affect		Responsiveness
1	*Facial* expression shows no emotion during the student's activities, praise/feedback and attention are absent, and attentive body language is absent.	1	*Does not* respond to the student's initiations, behavior, body language, and requests.
1.5	*Limited* emotion is shown, very little verbal praise/feedback or attention is given, and attentive body language is minimal.	1.5	Shows *limited/inconsistent* responses to the student's behavior, body language, and requests.
2	Attentive/expressive at times, and/or may give some verbal praise/feedback. Exhibits *some* attentive body language.	2	Is *somewhat* responsive to the student's initiations, behavior, body language, and requests in several instances. May have *neutral* response to student.
2.5	*Frequently* attentive and expressive, giving *frequent* verbal praise/feedback, and exhibiting positive/attentive body language the majority of the time.	2.5	*Frequently and positively* responds to the student's initiations, behavior, body language, and requests.
3	Positive praise/feedback and/or instruction is given in a calm or enthusiastic tone of voice, there are *several* instances of observable enjoyment with the student through positive attention and emotional facial expressions, & attentive body language is *continually* used.	3	Responds *consistently and positively* to the student's initiations, behavior, body language, and requests.

Teacher Engagement Rating Scale: Hints for Coding

<u>Level of Affect:</u> Measures the teacher's interest in/attention to the student or his/her activity.

1   The teacher appears disinterested in the student and his/her activities. The teacher may appear flat or show negative emotions toward student. The teacher does not show interest through his/her body language, such as sitting up, leaning forward, etc.
1.5   The teacher shows limited interest in the student and may briefly comment on his/her activity. Occasional praise/feedback may be given. The teacher does not interact positively with the student.
2   The teacher has neutral affect toward the student (is not angry with the student or ignoring them, but does not smile at them, etc.). Some praise/feedback is given and the teacher attends somewhat to the student.
2.5   The teacher frequently gives praise/feedback to the student and is interested in them. The teacher shows positive affect.
3   The teacher is enthusiastic about student/student's activities, or teacher is clearly attending to student/student's activity and interacting with the student in a calm, pleasant manner. Shared enjoyment between the student and the teacher is observed through facial expression and/or positive body language. Praise and/or feedback are given in a positive manner.

<u>Maintenance of Interaction:</u> Measures degree to which the teacher builds on the student's initiation and/or assists the student in using objects functionally.

1   The teacher does not attempt to use different approaches (physical, verbal, gestural prompts) to build upon interaction. The teacher does not ask questions or introduce new elements to keep the student engrossed in task. The teacher may allow the student to use an object inappropriately without attempting to demonstrate its proper use (i.e., allows the student to mouth ball w/o teaching him/her to roll it).
1.5   The teacher makes few attempts to help the student to be productive. The teacher may demonstrate an object's use a few times, but is not persistent in the demonstration. The teacher does not monitor the interaction closely or look for ways to build upon it.
2   The teacher may show the student how to roll ball, then watches as he/she mouths it and partially corrects student/shows the student how to be more functional with ball. The teacher asks a few questions about activity to expand the interaction.
2.5   The teacher frequently looks for ways to help the student expand the interaction and asks questions about play. Or the teacher frequently assists the student in using objects correctly.
3   The teacher expands interaction by introducing new elements into play/ activity (i.e., the teacher may have doll catch ball, may show the student how to stack blocks according to color, etc.) and gives the student the support he/she needs to be successful in interactions with objects (physical, verbal, gestural prompts or physical assistance). The teacher may consistently ask questions that keep the student engaged and monitors the quality of the interaction.

<u>Directiveness:</u> Measures degree to which the teacher gives commands and/or directs the student's immediate attention.

1   The teacher does not allow time for the student to respond to request before repeating request and makes constant commands (i.e., "Do this," "Look at this," "Come here," etc.). The teacher may redirect student's interest or focus. Teacher may direct behavior through gestures, repetitive commands, & physical prompting.
1.5   The teacher frequently gives the student commands and only briefly waits for the student's response.
2   The teacher somewhat tries to direct the student's attention through prompts and offers a little time before demanding that the student comply with request.

2.5 The teacher uses commands infrequently and may find alternate ways to redirect the student's attention. The teacher follows the student's lead and interest and only occasionally repeats prompts and demand's the student's immediate attention.

3 The teacher is able to follow the student's lead throughout and only refocuses attention when he/she becomes distracted. The teacher directs attention to a different topic only when focus of attention is not productive. The teacher gives the student adequate time to comply with request.

Responsiveness: Measures frequency and intensity of the teacher's reactions to student's initiation with actions or objects.

1 The teacher ignores the student's requests, behavior, body language, etc. The teacher does not follow the student's initiation and does not reciprocate interaction with the student.

1.5 The teacher's responses to the student are restricted and he/she may often ignore the student's behaviors.

2 The teacher responds appropriately to the student's initiations, but is neither enthusiastic nor apathetic about his/her initiations.

2.5 The teacher is mostly attentive to the student and is generally positive toward his/her initiations.

3 The teacher fully attends to the student's body language, requests, and/or behavior. The teacher responds to student's initiations with enthusiasm. The teacher follows the student's lead in initiations.

Initiation: Measures degree to which the teacher begins interaction with student.

1 The teacher makes no attempt to interact with the student.

1.5 The teacher is passive but makes a partial attempt to begin an interaction.

2 The teacher takes some initiative to interact with the student, and interactions are neutral.

2.5 The teacher makes several attempts to begin interactions with the student.

3 The teacher is persistent in attempting to begin interactions with the student. Even if the student does not respond, the teacher will continue to initiate. The teacher interacts positively with the student.

Level of Movement/Participation: Measures degree to which the teacher stays on the student's physical level.

1 The teacher does not move with the student. The teacher may remain standing while the student sits and the teacher does not transition with the student. The teacher does not take part in the student's activities.

1.5 The teacher may occasionally move with the student and get on his/her physical level. The teacher may participate somewhat.

2 The teacher is somewhat interactive with the student and sometimes sits beside them or follows them to another activity.

2.5 The teacher generally sits on the child's level and/or follows the child to new activity. Participation is frequently observed.

3 The teacher sits on the floor with the student and constantly readjusts position as the student transitions to a new activity.

Appendix L   Multiple Trials Data Sheet

Student's Name: _____

Skill/Behavior: _____

Criterion Level: _____ Prompt: (*circle*) I=Independent V=Verbal Vi=Visual
G=Gestural P=Physical

Instructions: In the section above, describe the skill/behavior, criterion level,* and circle the prompt(s) for the objective. Using the table below, for each trial, indicate if the student passed (p) or failed (f). Sum the total number of trials passed and administered. Divide the number passed by the number administered to obtain the percent passed.

Day																		
1																		
2																		
3																		
4																		
5																		
6																		
7																		
8																		
9																		
10																		
11																		
12																		
13																		
14																		
15																		
16																		
17																		
18																		
19																		
20																		
# trials																		
# passed																		
% passed																		

*See Table 5.2 in Chap. 5 for more on the components of a well-developed IEP objective.

Appendix M   Activity-Based Data Sheet

Student's Name:_____ Skill/Behavior:_____

Dates: _____ Criterion Level: _____

Coaching Session: _____Prompt: (circle) I=Independent V=Verbal
Vi=Visual G=Gestural P=Physical

Instructions: In the section above, describe the skill/behavior, criterion level,* and circle the prompt(s) for the objective. Using the table below, list the prompts used, tally the number of times the student demonstrated the skill at the criterion level (# passed), and tally the number of opportunities provided (# opportunities). For the bottom row, tally the total number of times passed and the total number of opportunities.

Day		M	T	W	TH	F	M	T	W	TH	F
Date											
Activities											
	Prompt										
	# Passed										
	# Opportunities										
	Prompt										
	# Passed										
	# Opportunities										
	Prompt										
	# Passed										
	# Opportunities										
	Prompt										
	# Passed										
	# Opportunities										
Total # Passed # Opportunities											

*See Table 5.2 in Chap. 5 for more on the components of a well-developed IEP objective.

Chapter 9
COMPASS Case Studies

Overview: Chap. 9 provides case study examples of the COMPASS consultation and coaching procedural steps for three children with autism spectrum disorder who vary by age, cognitive functioning level, verbal skill, and primary classroom placement.

In this chapter, we:

1. Provide a detailed case study using Steps A and B of the COMPASS Consultation Action Plan (Fig. 9.1) and the COMPASS Coaching Protocol for a preschool child who is nonverbal and has behavioral issues.
2. Present two abridged case studies; first, a second grader who is minimally verbal and who splits his time equally between the special education classroom and general education classroom, and second, a third grader who has age-appropriate language skills and is in the general education classroom for most of the day.

This chapter provides COMPASS consultation and coaching case studies for three students who vary in cognitive and language abilities. Although all share social and communication impairments, they also have unique strengths and challenges that must be taken into account in their personalized teaching plans.

The first case study, which follows a 5-year-old named Anthony, is an extended example of a complete COMPASS Consultation Action Plan and the four coaching sessions that followed. We provide the completed COMPASS Challenges and Supports Form for Caregivers and Teachers for Anthony, as well as the completed Goal Attainment Scale (GAS) Form and teaching objectives.

The second case study, of Ethan, is an abridged example. The joint summary form is not included, but the GAS Form and teaching objectives are. The third case study, of Gary, is also abridged. In this third example, we provide suggested actions for the reader to consider. We encourage the reader to consider what teaching strategies he or she would employ before reading what the consultant did.

It should become clear from these case examples that although the systematic approach outlined in this manual was followed, the consultant also allowed for

L.A. Ruble et al., *Collaborative Model for Promoting Competence and Success for Students with ASD*, DOI 10.1007/978-1-4614-2332-4_9, © Springer Science+Business Media, LLC 2012

flexibility, teacher-directed problem solving, and creativity. Even though no two teaching plans were identical in these case studies, evidence-based practices were applied within the context of the COMPASS framework.

Case Study 1: Anthony

Background Information

At the time of his COMPASS consultation, Anthony was a 5-year-old African American boy who was diagnosed with autism at age 2 by autism specialists located in a university-based tertiary diagnostic center. He attended an inclusive public school preschool program in an urban area of a midwestern state and received approximately 12 h a week of special education services under the educational eligibility of autism.

Anthony's parents were recently separated. Anthony resided with his biological mother, 2-year-old sister, and infant brother in the home of the maternal grandparents. His father was a cook in a restaurant, and his mother was unemployed outside the home.

Anthony's preschool special education teacher, Ms. Caudill, was a Caucasian female who had taught for 12 years. She had been in her current position for 5 years. She was certified to teach mild and moderate special education K-12. Although she had no formal or supervised coursework in autism, she had attended several professional conferences in autism such as a TEACCH training, a Picture Exchange Communication workshop, training on applied behavior analysis, social stories training, video modeling training, and numerous national conferences in early childhood education. She had also accessed informal training from various sources such as books, a behavioral consultant, and the Internet. At the time, she had both assessment and teaching experiences with a total of nine children with autism. She used visual schedules, structured work tasks, communication boards, sensory modulation strategies, and social stories for students with autism. She also used discrete trial training, structured teaching methods, and play-based/incidental teaching methods throughout the day. Discrete trial was conducted one-on-one across several sessions, and play-based methods were used in short sessions. Ms. Caudill reported that her strengths in working with students with autism included the ability to adhere to a program or plan, the use of a variety of ideas that drew from her wide repertoire of skills and experience with children who have a variety of disabilities, and her ability to analyze student behavior and data.

Ms. Caudill reported that it was a challenge to find time to schedule collaborative meetings for developing and implementing programs for her students with autism. Email was used for most information sharing. For parent communication, she used three methods: discussion during Anthony's drop-off time on a daily basis, home notes on a weekly basis or an occasional note or call from Anthony's mother, and discussion during the IEP annual meeting.

Table 9.1 COMPASS consultation action plan for students with autism

Step A—Activities prior to a COMPASS consultation (covered in Chap. 6)

1. Gather information about the student from consultant observations and from the caregiver and teacher reports using the COMPASS Challenges and Supports Form for Caregivers and Teachers
2. Complete COMPASS Challenges and Supports Joint Summary Form

Step B—Activities during a COMPASS consultation (covered in Chap. 7)

1. Discuss COMPASS Consultation Training Packet
2. Discuss COMPASS Consultation Joint Summary
3. Identify and come to consensus on three prioritized objectives and write measurable objectives
4. Develop COMPASS teaching plans for each measurable objective

Ms. Caudill reported that the most challenging aspects of working with a student with autism were "having cohesion across a team" and "providing consistency across team members." She felt that other school personnel needed to learn more about the importance of consistency for students with autism and how to interpret behavior as communication. In summary, she indicated that she would like more training in team building and developing work tasks for cognitive skill development for students with autism who had limited verbal skills.

Each step of the COMPASS Consultation Action Plan is described below. Also, Table 9.1 illustrates the entire process for the action plan.

Step A. Activities Prior to a COMPASS Consultation

Step A. 1. Gather Information about the Student Using COMPASS Challenges and Supports Form for Caregivers and Teachers

Anthony's mother and teacher completed the COMPASS Challenges and Supports Form for Caregivers and Teachers. In addition to these forms, other assessment information was gathered using standardized and criterion-based tools.

Information from Direct Evaluation

Anthony completed standardized cognitive and language assessment conducted by the consultant in the classroom. Observational data also were collected on Anthony's learning and work behavior skills. His teacher thought that Anthony would be better able to complete tasks in a familiar environment. Despite this assumption, Anthony had difficulty throughout the assessment. He required physical prompting, verbal cuing, and environmental arrangement (i.e., placing his table in the corner away from distractions) to complete tasks. He tried repeatedly to escape from the chair and vocalized sounds (grunts) of refusal. He often pushed items away. His teacher remained close and assisted with reminders and verbal cues to Anthony. Eventually, work-reward routines were established and his engagement in tasks improved.

Test results revealed a standardized score (SS) of 50 for General Conceptual Ability (i.e., cognitive functioning) using the Differential Abilities Scale; and a SS of 68 for Listening Comprehension and 53 for Oral Expression using the Oral and Written Language Scales. Adaptive behavior reported by his teacher indicated a SS of 52 for Communication, 40 for Daily Living Skills, 56 for Socialization, and 62 for Motor Skills based on the Vineland-II. In summary, all of Anthony's test scores fell within the significantly below average range (more than two standard deviations below the mean) based on standardized test results. These findings indicate that in addition to autism, Anthony also has comorbid intellectual disability.

Two autism-specific instruments were also used to obtain additional information on social and communication skill development specific to autism. The Childhood Autism Rating Scale (CARS) was used to gather information on the severity of autism. The Autism Diagnostic Observation Schedule (ADOS) was also used to gather information on Anthony's communication, social, and play skills. The CARS indicated a score of 38, suggesting moderate-to-severe autism. The ADOS scale for communication indicated a lack of vocalizations directed to others and use of gestures. He did use a sign for "more," but he did not look toward the person. For social interaction, he did not make eye contact with others or direct facial expressions toward others. He also did not show items to share enjoyment in interactions or initiate any joint attention with the examiner. He did follow the examiner's pointing gesture toward a toy and tried to imitate by pointing as well. For play skills, he played functionally with cause and effect toys and pretended to give a doll a drink from a cup. Stereotyped behaviors were also observed as he showed hand and finger mannerisms. It was difficult to obtain his interest to attend to objects and he became distressed if preferred objects were removed.

Criterion-based assessment was used to obtain descriptions of Anthony's learning skills. The Learning Skills Checklist (item 8 available in the COMPASS Challenges and Supports Form for Caregivers and Teachers of Chap. 6) indicated that the following skills were emerging (he could do with some cues/prompts, but not independently) for Anthony: (a) ability to understand the concept of "finished;" (b) recognize and indicate a need for help; (c) indicate to another that he is finished; (d) understand "rewards" as a consequence of work; (e) understand the concept of "wait;" (f) refocus attention in face of distractions; (f) initiate work and play activities; (g) perform tasks involving multiple materials; (h) use trial and error; and (i) use self-correction. The only skill he failed to demonstrate was the ability to work independently for short periods.

Observation of Anthony's engagement-related behaviors as he was being instructed by his teacher was completed using the Autism Engagement Rating Scale in Chap. 8. Engagement with his teacher was quite discrepant compared to his behaviors with the evaluator. The observation with his teacher indicated that he was frequently cooperative and attentive to the activities. He functionally used some, but not all, tools or objects. He required some prompts (verbal, gestural, and physical) to complete tasks throughout the activity. For the most part, there was consistency between the teacher's goals and Anthony's goals during the instruction. In other words, both were focused on the same activity, and Anthony was not attending to another object or activity in the classroom.

Step A. 2. Complete COMPASS Challenges and Supports Joint Summary Form

The COMPASS Challenges and Supports Form for Caregivers and Teachers was completed by his parents and teacher separately. They were collected and summarized into a single document using the COMPASS Challenges and Supports Joint Summary Form prior to the COMPASS consultation, which is replicated later in this chapter. Anthony's mother had not completed all the forms prior to the consultation, thus information was collected as the consultation ensued. This is not typical, but does happen on occasion and the consultant needs to be able to respond flexibly when unanticipated issues arise. The information provided and also collected during the consultation was reviewed during Step B of COMPASS consultation.

Step B: Activities During a COMPASS Consultation

Step B. 1. Discuss COMPASS Consultation Training Packet

A. Introductions and Sign In

At the consultation were Anthony's teacher, a teaching assistant, his mother, and the consultant. Introductions were made and the purpose and outcomes of the COMPASS consultation were described. Each member received two packets used during the consult. The first packet, the COMPASS Consultation Training Packet, provided information on the overview of the COMPASS model, explanation of best practices, expected outcomes from the consultation, and forms to create the COMPASS balance between challenges and supports and a teaching plan. The second packet was the summarized information (COMPASS Challenges and Supports Joint Summary Form) collected from both Anthony's teacher and parents.

B. Explanation of COMPASS

The instructions for completing Step B of COMPASS Consultation Action Plan provided in Chap. 7 were followed. The Abridged Protocol for Step B of the COMPASS Consultation Action Plan and scripts provided in the forms section were copied and used as a guide by the consultant during the consultation.

C. Explanation of Purpose/Outcomes of COMPASS Consultation

After the COMPASS model was explained, the next steps of covering the specific purpose of the consultation and expected outcomes were provided using the scripts.

D. Overview of Best Practices

An explanation of best practices was presented next. Little interaction between the consultant and participants took place up to this point. Most of the information was shared one-way and was intended to set up the next discussion activity. The consultant did check in with the participants and ask if they had any questions as information was presented.

Step B. 2. Discuss COMPASS Challenges and Supports Joint Summary Form

Next, the COMPASS Challenges and Supports Joint Summary Form was provided to each participant (see page 192). The consultant made notes on comments provided by Anthony's mom and teacher as the information was reviewed. The discussion clarified areas of concern, brought out strengths, and generally contributed to everyone's better understanding of how Anthony engaged at home, school, and in the community.

The discussion began with a review of Anthony's strengths and interests. The consultant used this information to remind the participants that Anthony has several personal protective factors and supports that can be used to reinforce and motivate him. Overall, he enjoys music and singing. He seeks tactile input such as hugs, deep touches, and rough play. He enjoys rocking, swinging, and running. His mother reported that he can be "obsessive" with small animals, and this interest can interfere with activities at home, however. His mother also reported that he has relative strengths in responding to and engaging in joint attention with adults. Another significant strength for Anthony is the ability to identify pictures. He uses pictures to understand work routines and the daily schedule.

In review of Anthony's personal challenges, many issues were noted with personal management and adaptive behavior skills. Areas marked with a "3" or "4" denoted significant challenges. Several behaviors were marked as concerns by his mother and teacher within the areas of adaptive skills. Fears and frustrations were noted and included going to new places as well as being told "no" for a desired request. His teacher also noted that being asked to complete a new task he did not understand frustrated him.

Most notable during the consultation was the report from his teacher and parent on the frequency, severity, and intensity of problem behavior. His teacher reported that he aggressed toward others more than 12 times daily on average. Hitting occurred, but not as much as pinching. The problem behaviors were so severe that his teachers and teaching assistants were concerned about the safety of the other students in the classroom and therefore felt that an adult needed to be by him at all times. The consultant made notes about this information and refrained from offering suggestions because the aim of this part of the consultation process was sharing information, not problem solving. Problem solving takes place following the identification of prioritized teaching objectives. The consultant did make notes to come back to this issue. Also, the consultant mentally noted that as a consequence of the problem behaviors, Anthony's development of pivotal skills was hindered. He had reduced opportunities to be independent and to learn how to interact with other children in the classroom.

A review of the teacher- and parent-reported social skills indicated that Anthony had weaknesses in most areas of imitating, turn-taking, joint attention, and playing. Most social interactions involving children were weak. Due to behavioral concerns, his teacher and teaching assistants were concerned about him interacting and being in close proximity to his classroom peers. The consultant made notes on these concerns so that social skills, as replacement skills for aggression, would be discussed and included as a priority in the teaching plan.

A review of Anthony's communication means and functions indicated that he used physical means to communicate all messages. He was essentially nonverbal, and instead took adults to the objects and activities he desired. To express refusals, confusion, and feelings of anger, he yelled, hit, and scratched and occasionally shook his head "no." He used a picture to communicate when he was finished. The consultant helped the participants understand the connection between his problem behaviors and lack of communication skills. The consultant made notes to ensure that communication skills related to requests and refusals would be addressed as a priority.

Anthony's responses to sensory input in his environment revealed areas of agreement, but also differences between school and home report, which is to be expected. He had particular issues with auditory, tactile, taste, and vestibular input. He feared some noises and was distracted by others. He had many tactile sensitivities reported by his teacher that included mouthing objects. Eating was a major issue. He had limited food preferences such as chicken nuggets, pretzels, chips, and sausage. He did eat bananas and apples.

Anthony's learning skills were discussed. His teacher reported that he did not start or complete any tasks independently. Often when presented with an undesired task, he aggressed. His teacher created a choice board from which he could choose what work activities he would complete. The consultant reminded the participants that if Anthony did have the ability to start and complete undesired tasks, then problem behaviors would decrease. The consultant made notes to ensure that learning skills be discussed as a priority skills.

At the conclusion of reviewing the joint summary information, the consultant reviewed the concerns listed at the start of the consultation and considered them against the information just reviewed. Anthony's mother and teacher both reported concerns with peer interactions and aggression. Anthony's teacher also reported issues with developing adaptive and independent skills. All concerns reported by Anthony's teacher and mother confirmed the issues brought out using the joint summary form and noted by the consultant. The next section provides the discussion on how consensus was achieved regarding parent and teacher concerns.

Case Study 1: Anthony

COMPASS Challenges and Supports Joint Summary Form

1. Student's Likes, Strengths, Frustrations and Fears

Likes/Preferences/Interests:

	Teacher:	Caregiver:
Activities:	• Music • Art activities • Singing familiar songs	• Music and singing
Objects/Toys:	• Farm animals/animals • Will look at a book briefly if • about animals	• Animals (obsessed with them)

Strengths or abilities

Teacher:	Caregiver:
• Lovable, shows affection • Memory! He never forgets some things • Learns new tasks quickly • Good eye contact to familiar adults • Watches—really observant • Receptive vocabulary is a relative strength • Good gross motor skills	

Frustrations

Teacher:	Caregiver:

• Anthony has difficulty communicating why he is
  frustrated
• He gets very angry when he is denied a want, is not
  allowed to change his schedule or have an item, or does not
  understand a task	

Fears

Teacher:	Caregiver:
• Not sure on this one • New situations either excite him or make him anxious • Sometimes loud noises upset him	• New, unfamiliar places

2. Adaptive Skills

These skills were marked as very difficult.

Personal Management	Teacher	Caregiver
Performing basic self care independently (such as toileting, dressing, eating, using utensils)	X	X
Entertaining self in free time		
Changing activities—transitioning	X	X. Varies daily
Sleeping		
Comments: Anthony used to be transported in a wagon due to running off. He does not go anywhere without holding hands. Any change causes him to be upset. Tool use is a problem and most things go in his mouth.		
Responding to others	Teacher	Caregiver
Following 1 or 2 step direction	X	X
Accepting "no"	X	X
Answering questions	X	X
Accepting help		
Accepting correction	X	X
Being quiet when required	X	
Comments: He can respond to simple directions.		
Understanding group behaviors	Teacher	Caregiver
Coming when called to group	X	
Staying within certain places—lines, circles, chairs, desks	X	X
Participating with the group	X	
Talking one at a time		
Picking up, cleaning up, straightening up, putting away		
Comments: When he initiates to come to group, he does not tantrum. Staying in certain places is improving. At Walmart or Kroger, he has to be in shopping cart for fear of running off. He may tremble if at a new place due to fear.		
Understanding community expectations	Teacher	Caregiver
Understanding who is a stranger	X	X
Going to places in the community (place of worship, stores, restaurants, malls, homes)	X	X Doesn't go
Understanding safety (such as streets, seatbelts)	X	X
Managing transportation (Cars/buses)	X	X. Doesn't go
Comments: His mom reports that these are very vague concepts for him.		

3. Problem Behaviors*

These behaviors were marked as problematic.

		Teacher	Caregiver
1.	Acting impulsively, without thinking	X	X
2.	Hitting or hurting others	X	X
3.	Damaging or breaking things that belong to others	X	X
4.	Screaming or yelling	X	X
5.	Having sudden mood changes	X	X
6.	Having temper tantrums	X	X
7.	Having a low frustration tolerance; becoming easily angered or upset	X	X
8.	Crying easily		
9.	Being overly quiet, shy, or withdrawn		
10.	Acting sulky or sad		
11.	Being underactive or lacking in energy		
12.	Engaging in behaviors that may be distasteful to others, such as nose-picking or spitting		
13.	Touching him/herself inappropriately		
14.	Engaging in compulsive behaviors; repeating certain acts over and over		
15.	Hitting or hurting him/herself		
16.	Becoming overly upset when others touch or move his/her belongings		
17.	Laughing/giggling at inappropriate times (e.g., when others are hurt or upset)		
18.	Ignoring or walking away from others during interactions or play		
19.	Touching others inappropriately		
20.	Engaging in unusual mannerisms such as hand-flapping or spinning	X	X
21.	Having to play or do things in the same exact way each time		
22.	Having difficulty calming him/herself down when upset or excited	X	X
23.	Other: _____		

*Items are based on the Triad Social Skills Assessment

4. Social Skills (S = strength; W = weakness)

How well does the child:

		With adults		With children	
		Teacher	Caregiver	Teacher	Caregiver
Social awareness					
1.	Look toward a person who is talking to him/her	S	W	S	W
2.	Accept others being close to him/her	S	S	S	W
3.	Watch people for extended periods of time	W	W	W	S
4.	Respond to another person's approach by smiling or vocalizing	S	S	S	W
5.	Initiate interactions for social reasons	W	W	W	W
Joint attention skills					
6.	Look at something another person points to	S	S	W	W
7.	Show something to a person and look for person's reaction	W	W	W	W
8.	Point at an object or event to direct another person's attention to share enjoyment	S	S	W	W
9.	Share smile by looking back and forth between object and person	W	W	W	W
Imitation					
10.	Imitate sounds another person makes	S	W	S	W
11.	Imitate what another person does with an object (e.g., person makes toy airplane fly, child repeats action)	S	S	S	W
12.	Imitate body movements of others (such as, clap when others clap, play Simon Says)	S	S	S	W
13.	Imitate and expand upon other's actions with toys (e.g., peer beats drum, child beats drum and also starts to march)	S	NR	W	W
Play					
14.	Take turns within familiar routines (e.g., rolls a ball back and forth)	W	W	W	W
15.	Share toys	W	W	W	W
16.	Play interactively around a common theme	W	W	W	W
17.	Repair breakdowns during interactions (such as, child repeats or changes own behavior when other person seems confused or ignores)	S	W	S	W
18.	Pretends to do something or be something (such as, that a plate is a hat by putting it on, to be a policeman, to have a tea party, that a doll is a teacher)	W	W	W	W

5. Communication Skills

The following are descriptions of words or actions your child/student uses to communicate:

Making requests	Teacher	Caregiver
1. Food	Takes you by the hand; gets it himself	Mom agreed with teacher for most messages
2. Objects	Takes adult to area where object is	Often just gets it
3. An activity	Takes adult to where activity occurs	May just do it, like go outside to play
4. To use the toilet	Does not indicate or show awareness of	Does not do
5. Attention	Not sure; he seldom appears to want attention	May climb in my lap
6. Help	Uses a picture; needs to be prompted	Whines
7. To play	Takes object	Does by himself
8. Information	Does not request information	Does not do
9. A choice	Does not do	Does not do
Expressing refusals	Teacher	Caregiver
1. "Go away"	Yells, hits, scratches	Yells, hits, scratches
2. "No, I won't do it" or "I don't want it"	Yells, hits, scratches, occasionally signs "NO"	Yells, hits, scratches, occasionally signs "NO"
3. "I want to be finished" or "I want to stop doing this"	Same as question 1, is beginning to touch finished picture	Does not do
Expressing thoughts	Teacher	Caregiver
1. Greeting to others	Does not do	May look
2. Comments about people/environment	Does not do	Does not do
3. Confusion or "I don't know"	Yells, hits, bites, scratches if confused	Yells, hits, bites, scratches if confused
4. Comments about errors or things wrong	Does not do	Does not do
5. Asks about past/future event	Does not do	Does not do
6. Agreement	Takes object	Takes object
Expressing feelings	Teacher	Caregiver
1. Angry/mad/frustrated	Yells, slaps hits, bites	Yells, slaps hits, bites
2. Pain, illness, or hurt	Yells, slaps hits, bites	Have to guess
3. Happy/excited	Smiles	Will laugh and jump
4. Hurt feelings/upset	Yells, hits, slaps	Yells, hits, slaps
5. Afraid	Same as question 4; cries, cowers	Trembles
6. Sad	Same as question 4; does cry but as part of a tantrum	Cries

Comments: Pinching is reduced this year and he is scratching instead. He may also throw himself on the ground.

6. Sensory Challenges

These items were identified as being applicable to your child/student:

Sound/Auditory	Teacher	Caregiver
Has been diagnosed with hearing problem at some time	☐	☐
Reacts to unexpected sounds	☐	☒
Fears some noises	☒	☒
Distracted by certain sounds	☐	☐
Confused about direction of sounds	☐	☐
Makes self-induced noises	☒	☐
Fails to listen or pay attention to what is said to him/her	☐	☐
Talks a great deal	☐	☐
Own talking interferes with listening	☐	☐
Overly sensitive to some sounds	☐	☐
Seeks out certain noises or sounds	☐	☐
Other:_____	☐	☐

Taste	Teacher	Caregiver
Has an eating problem	☒	☒
Dislikes certain foods and textures	☒	☒
Will only eat a small variety of foods	☒	☒
Tastes/eats nonedibles	☒	☒
Explores environment by tasting	☒	☒
Puts most things in his/her mouth	☒	☒
Constant chewing on something	☐	☐
Other: can't have milk; lactose intolerant; does not eat sugars; eats chicken nuggets; grain cereal; sausage; pretzels; chips; banana/apple; drinks apple juice and water.	☒	☒

Sight/Vision	Teacher	Caregiver
Has trouble discriminating shapes, colors	☐	☐
Is sensitive to light—squints, wants to wear hats or sunglasses	☐	☐
Has trouble following with eyes	☐	☐
Does not make much eye contact	☐	☐
Is distracted by some or too much visual stimuli	☒	☐
Becomes excited when confronted with a variety of visual stimuli	☒	☐
Dislikes having eyes covered	☐	☐
Excited by vistas and open spaces	☒	☐
Hesitates going up or down stairs, curbs, or climbing equipment	☐	☐
Upset by things looking different (spills, spots)	☐	☐
Makes decisions about food, clothing, objects by sight	☐	☐
Closely examines objects or hands	☐	☐
Wants environment in certain order	☐	☐
Other:_____	☐	☐

(continued)

(continued)

Touch/Tactile	Teacher	Caregiver
Has to know someone is going to touch ahead of time	☐	☐
Dislikes being held or cuddled	☐	☐
Seems irritated when touched or bumped by peers	☐	☐
Explores environment by touching objects	☒	☐
Dislikes the feel of certain clothing	☐	☐
Refuses to touch certain things	☒	☐
Over or under dresses for the temperature or is unaware of temperature	☐	☐
	☐	☐
Doesn't like showers or rain on self	☒	☐
Mouths objects or clothing	☐	☐
Refuses to walk on certain surfaces	☐	☐
Dislikes having hair, face, or mouth touched	☐	☐
Upset by sticky, gooey hands	☐	☐
Touches items with feet before hands	☐	☐
Doesn't like to hold hands	☒	☐
Pinches, bites, or hurts himself	☐	☐
Other:_____		

Smell/Olfactory	Teacher	Caregiver
Sensitive to smells	☐	☐
Smells objects, food, people, toys more than usual	☐	☐
Explores environment by smelling	☐	☐
Reacts defensively to some smells	☐	☐
Ignores strong odors	☐	☐
Seeks out certain odors	☐	☐
Other:_____	☐	☐

Movement/Vestibular	Teacher	Caregiver
Seems fearful in space (teeter-totter, climbing)	☐	☐
Arches back when held or moved	☒	☒
Spins or whirls self around	☒	☒
Moves parts of body a great deal	☐	☐
Walks on toes	☒	☒
Appears clumsy, bumping into things and falling down	☐	☐
Avoids balance activities	☐	☐
Doesn't like to be around people in motion	☐	☐
Bumps into things and/or people	☐	☐
Other:_poor balance_____	☒	☐

Visual/Perceptual motor	Teacher	Caregiver
Has trouble with paper/pencil activities	☐	☐
Has difficulty with time perception	☐	☐
Has difficulty with body in space—moving appropriately	☐	☐
Has problems with use of some tools	☒	☒
Has problems organizing materials and moving them appropriately	☐	☐
Is distracted by doors and cupboards being open, holes, or motion	☐	☐
Other:_____	☐	☐

7. Sensory Supports

These items were identified as being applicable to your child/student:

Sound/Auditory	Teacher	Caregiver
Likes music	☒	☒
Likes to sing and dance	☒	☒
Taste	Teacher	Caregiver
Has definite eating preferences	☒	☐
Other:_____	☐	☐
Sight/Vision	Teacher	Caregiver
Enjoys watching moving things/bright objects	☒	☐
Enjoys patterns or shiny surfaces	☒	☒
Likes TV, videos, video games	☐	☐
Likes the computer	☒	☐
Other:_____	☐	☐
Touch/Tactile	Teacher	Caregiver
Likes to be touched	☒	☐
Likes hugs and cuddling when he/she initiates it	☒	☐
Likes to play in water	☒	☐
Likes baths or swimming pools	☐	☐
Seeks out mud, sand, clay to touch	☐	☐
Prefers deep touching rather than soft	☐	☐
Prefers certain textures of clothing	☐	☐
Likes being rolled or sandwiched between blankets/cushions	☐	☐
Likes rough and tumble play	☒	☐
Other:_____	☐	☐
Movement/Vestibular	Teacher	Caregiver
Enjoys rocking, swinging, spinning	☒	☐
Likes being tossed in the air	☐	☐
Likes to run	☒	☐
Likes and needs to move	☒	☐
Likes to climb; seldom falls	☒	☐
Other: __poor balance_____	☒	☐
Visual/Perceptual motor	Teacher	Caregiver
Relies on knowing location of furniture, stationary objects	☐	☐
Likes to draw and reproduce figures	☐	☐
Other:_____	☐	☐

8. Learning Skills

Learning/Work skill		Teacher	Caregiver
1.	Child clearly understands the end goal of an activity, recognize what he/she must do to be finished, and persists on the task to completion	W	W
2.	Child realizes when he/she is running into difficulty and has some way of letting the adult know he/she needs help	W	W
3.	Once an activity is under way, the adult can walk away from the child and he/she will keep working until finished, maintaining at least fairly good attention to what he/she is doing	W	W
4.	Child finishes work and remembers on his/her own to let the adult know (e.g., by bringing work to adult, calling adult, raising his/her hand)	W	W
5.	Child looks forward to earning a reward, knows it's next, works toward it, may ask for it or go get it on his/her own when work is finished	W	W
6.	Child is able to wait briefly for a direction (anticipates that he/she is about to be asked to do something), is able to wait briefly for his/her turn with a toy (anticipating that it's about to return him/her), and/or wait for something to happen	W	W
7.	Child may be distracted by outside sights and sounds or inner distractions (evident perhaps in singing to him/herself, gazing off, lining up materials) but is able to refocus attention to work on his/her own after a short time and without a prompt or reminder from the adult	W	W
8.	Child shows interest in and curiosity about materials, handles them without prompting or nudging from the adult to get started. When one activity is finished he/she will look for another	W	W
9.	Child can organize his/her responses to perform tasks when multiple materials are in front of him/her (e.g., a stack of cards for sorting)	W	W
10.	Child recognizes when one strategy is not working and tries another way	W	W
11.	Child recognizes his/her own mistakes and goes back and corrects them (e.g., takes little peg out of big hole to make room for correct peg)	W	W

9. Environmental Challenges

Describe challenges noted in the Forms or reported during the consultation:

- ☐ Behavioral/Knowledge/Attitude of Other People Variables (e.g., inability to communicate clearly to the student, teach skills necessary for the activity, establish positive work or play routines).
  - • Teaching assistants lack training.
- ☐ Procedural/Organizational (e.g., noisy environments, lack of visual supports, lack of effective transition routines).
  - • Lots of auditory and visual distractions in the classrooms.
  - • Lack of consistency between home and school.
- ☐ Temporal (e.g., lack or ineffective use of visual supports to understand passage of time or when activity is finished).
- ☐ Spatial (e.g., lack of personal space or clear boundaries).
  - • Relatively large classroom of students.
- ☐ Other
  - • Living in temporary and less familiar setting.
  - • Parents experiencing conflict and are stressed.
  - • A lot of unstructured time at home.
  - • New baby brother.
  - • Lacks involvement in community activities outside home.
  - • Does not receive any in-home services.
  - • There is limited time for the teacher to plan with teaching assistants.

10. Environmental Supports

Describe environmental supports of the child/student. Environmental supports are factors that facilitate learning. Examples are positive routines, use of rewards, and use of visuals supports.

- □ Behavioral/Knowledge/Attitude of other people variables (e.g., is able to communicate clearly to the student, teach skills necessary for the activity, establish positive work or play routines).

  - Teacher with a lot of specialized training in autism.
  - Many sociable peers in his classroom.
  - Teacher who likes to use technology and who has expressed desire to learn more about teaching methods.

- □ Procedural/Organizational (e.g., uncluttered environments, visual supports for understanding work routines, positive transition routines).

  - Teacher who uses a lot of visual supports, including signs and gestures, to communicate.
  - Teacher uses visual schedules and pictures to help understand and to communicate with others.
  - Teacher who builds choice into Anthony's activities.
  - Teacher who knows Anthony well and knows what motivates and frustrates him.

- □ Temporal (e.g., visual supports to understand passage of time or when activity is finished).

  - Teacher uses visual schedules and pictures to help understand the order of events.

- □ Spatial (e.g., personal space to work and calm down, clear boundaries).
- □ Other

  - Teacher and mother who desire the same outcomes for Anthony.
  - Mother who is seeking a more permanent living situation.

11. Summary of Concerns

<u>Social and play skills</u>

Teacher	Caregiver
1. "Normalized" play routines: move away from repetitive and self-stimulating type of play	1. Interacting with peers.
2. Increase appropriate peer interactions	2.

<u>Communication skills</u>

Teacher	Caregiver
1. Express emotions without hurting others	1.
2.	2.

<u>Learning skills</u>

Teacher	Caregiver
1. Completing requested tasks	1.
2. Independent work: only works with adult direction at the time	2.

<u>Adaptive skills</u>

Teacher	Caregiver
1. Personal care routines: would like to see Anthony gain more independence	1.
2.	2.

<u>Other (if there is another area)</u>

Teacher	Caregiver
1. Controlling temper	1. Anger
2.	2.

Step B. 3. Identify and Come to Consensus on Three Prioritized Objectives and Write Measurable Objectives

After the joint summary and parent and teacher priorities were reviewed in detail, three teaching objectives were identified. The consultant reminded the participants that a goal of the COMPASS consultation was to identify a social skill, a work or learning skill, and a communication skill to teach. The consultant also reminded the teacher and mother that often there is agreement in what they both report, but that sometimes there was disagreement and that this is expected. School settings are very structured and sometimes children respond very well to this structure. But at the same time, while home is less structured, children might respond better there. The differences in reporting are considered valid observations because children

Table 9.2 Anthony's COMPASS/IEP objectives

1. When presented with a task menu, Anthony will start and complete three 2-3 minute tasks each day without aggression with one adult verbal cue (e.g., time to work) and gestural/picture cues across 2 weeks

2. During structured play, Anthony will imitate adult play activities for five actions (actions with objects) with at least three different preferred objects (dinosaurs, animals, doll) each day across 2 weeks

3. Anthony will make 10 different requests per day independently (go home, eat, help, more, finished, various objects/activities) or as a response to a question ("what do you want?") using sign, pictures, or verbalization on a daily basis for 2 weeks

with autism respond differently at home and at school. When there are significant differences, issues of generalization might be discussed. In the case of Anthony, the reader will notice that the teacher was a better observer/reporter compared to his mother. Sometimes this is the case, but usually not.

Because of Anthony's aggression, much discussion followed about the underlying reasons and purposes of his behavior problems and the parents' and teacher's main concern about aggression. The consultant reviewed the concept of replacement skills to help Anthony's teacher and parent understand that with better work skills, communication skills, and social interaction skills, Anthony's aggression will reduce.

The iceberg illustration in the COMPASS Consultation Training Packet was used to facilitate this discussion. At the tip of the iceberg, descriptions of Anthony's aggressive behaviors were written. These included hitting, pinching, and slapping. Below the iceberg, the team hypothesized reasons for the aggression. To help develop reasons for aggression, his communication skills were reviewed again to remind participants of the importance of identifying the communicative functions of behavior. Three primary functions were hypothesized: (a) wanting a desired activity or object and being told "no;" (b) wanting to be finished with an undesired activity; and (c) refusing to start an activity. Anthony's personal challenges included lack of negotiation skills that stem from communication problems and a lack of understanding the impact of his problem behaviors on others. A lack of motivation to "please" others was also discussed as a contributor to the aggression. At the same time, as objectives designed to reduce behavior were discussed, the consultant encouraged the team to consider skills to be enhanced. As a result, objectives that focused on starting and completing a task, initiating a variety of requests, and interacting with peers by increasing play skills were discussed as potential prosocial and replacement skills for aggression. After much discussion, the replacement skills and teaching objectives in Table 9.2 were identified and written as measurable IEP objectives. Information on how to write measurable objectives is provided in Chap. 5.

Developing the Goal Attainment Scale

After the objectives were written in measurable terms, they were then added to the GAS Form. Recall from Chap. 8 that the GAS Form is used to facilitate progress monitoring as the teaching plans were implemented. Anthony's present levels of performance were described at the −2 level for each of the three objectives. Next, the objective as written for goal attainment was placed at the 0 level. This was the skill he was expected to achieve by the end of the school year. Measurable increments of behavioral change were noted at levels −1, +1, and +2. Notice that the items that are in parentheses denote how the skill level may vary, and that if the child meets expectations noted in at least one area denoted by the parenthesis, progress is made at that level. For example, Anthony is expected to be able to start and complete three 2–3 min tasks each day without aggression with one adult verbal cue (e.g., time to work) and gestural/picture cues across 2 weeks by the end of the school year. If he is making progress toward this skill, he may be able to complete one (as indicated in the parentheses) instead of three tasks with no aggression or need two (as indicated in the parentheses) instead of one verbal cue to start. If he is able to accomplish the goal, but with fewer work items or more cues, then he is above baseline and is making progress.

Goal Attainment Scale Form for Anthony

−2 Present level of performance	−1 Progress	0 Expected level of outcome (GOAL)	+1 Somewhat more than expected	+2 Much more than expected
Aggresses when given a task he does not want to do. Is difficult to motivate. Does not have a more appropriate way to communicate refusals or to negotiate	When presented with a task menu, Anthony will start and complete three (1) 2–3 min tasks each day without aggression with one (2) adult verbal cue (e.g., time to work) and gestural/ picture cues across 2 weeks	When presented with a task menu, Anthony will start and complete three 2–3 min tasks each day without aggression with one adult verbal cue (e.g., time to work) and gestural/picture cues across 2 weeks	When presented with a task menu, Anthony will start and complete three (4) 2–3 min tasks each day without aggression with one (0) adult verbal cue (e.g., time to work) and gestural/ picture cues across 2 weeks	When presented with a task menu, Anthony will start and complete three (6) 2–3 min tasks each day without aggression with one (0) adult verbal cue (e.g., time to work) and gestural/ picture cues across 2 weeks
Has difficulty imitating others, especially children using actions with objects. Likes objects he can manipulate	Anthony will imitate play activities for five (2) minutes with at least three (1) different preferred objects (dinosaurs, animals, doll ...) each day across 2 weeks	Anthony will imitate adult play activities for 5 min with at least three different preferred objects (dinosaurs, animals, doll...) each day across 2 weeks	Anthony will imitate adult play activities for five (7) minutes with at least three (4) different preferred objects (dinosaurs, animals, doll ...) each day across 2 weeks	Anthony will imitate adult (peer) play activities for five (10) minutes with at least three (6) differ- ent preferred objects (dinosaurs, animals, doll ...) each day across 2 weeks

(continued)

(continued)

−2 Present level of performance	−1 Progress	0 Expected level of outcome (GOAL)	+1 Somewhat more than expected	+2 Much more than expected
May use aggression as a way to request. Relies on adult prompts to make requests	Anthony will make 10 (5) different requests per day independently (with verbal cues) or as a response to a question (go home, eat, help, more, finished, various objects/ activities) using sign, pictures, or verbal on a daily basis for 2 weeks	Anthony will make 10 different requests per day independently (go home, eat, help, more, finished, various objects/ activities) or as a response to a question ("what do you want?") using sign, pictures, or verbalization on a daily basis for 2 weeks	Anthony will make 10 (15) different requests per day independently (go home, eat, help, more, finished, various objects/ activities) or as a response to a question ("what do you want?") using sign, pictures, or verbalization on a daily basis for 2 weeks	Anthony will make 10 (20) different requests per day independently (go home, eat, help, more, finished, various objects/ activities) or as a response to a question ("what do you want?") using sign, pictures, or verbalization on a daily basis for 2 weeks

Step B. 4. Develop COMPASS Teaching Plans for each Measurable Objective

Depending on the amount of time necessary for completing steps 2 and 3, adjustments may need to be made for completing step 4 of the COMPASS Consultation Action Plan. For Anthony's consultation, because a significant amount of time was required to identify the replacement skills for aggression and to develop the objectives, little time was left for developing teaching plans for the second and third skills during the time allocated for the consultation. As a result, the consultant asked the teacher to work on the teaching plans and those not finished or unclear were completed at the first coaching session.

For each objective, the team identified Anthony's personal and environmental challenges that would hinder attainment of the skill and identified Anthony's personal and environmental supports to consider for teaching the skill and adding to his teaching plan. The three objectives and teaching plans are outlined below.

Teaching Plan for Objective 1

Objective 1: When presented with a task menu, Anthony will start and complete three 2-3 min tasks each day without aggression with one adult verbal cue (e.g., time to work) and gestural/picture cues across 2 weeks.

Personal and Environmental Challenges and Supports for Teaching Plan 1

Personal challenges	*Environmental challenges*
• Uses aggression to communicate many wants/needs/refusals, including confusion • Has low expressive language skills • Has limited repertoire of preferred tasks—most work tasks are unpreferred • Lacks motivation to please others • Lacks motivation for many objects/activities	• Is in an integrated setting with a lot of other students • Has many physical distractions in the environment • Has living arrangements at home that have changed and are a bit unstable • Has new baby brother at home
Personal supports	*Environmental supports*
• Likes animals and small animal toys he can hold in his hand • Has better receptive compared to expressive language skills • Understands many pictures • Uses a picture to indicate being finished consistently	• Has mother and teacher who want same outcomes • Has teacher and assistant who know Anthony well • See teaching plan for specific supports and strategies to teach this skill

The teaching plan for objective 1 developed with the team is below:

Teaching Plan

1. Review the Evidence-based Online Resources for Teachers in the forms section of Chap. 7, in particular those on structured work systems and structured teaching.
2. Develop and keep current a task menu that indicates to Anthony his work tasks. Be sure these are tasks he is familiar with and can do independently.
3. For each work task, have a visual task analysis (pictures) that displays each step of the task or have the tasks structured so he knows what to do. Provide visual cues of how much work he is to do or how he is to know when he is finished (i.e., sort the cars by color until they are all in the right bowls).
4. Refer to videos of structured teaching methods available online at: http://www.autisminternetmodules.org/user_mod.php and at http://autismpdc.fpg.unc.edu/content/structured-work-systems.
5. Begin with short work tasks with a learned visual that represents the work task and a visual that shows the reward he will receive following the work task.
6. For the rewards, gather items and place in a basket (due to low motivation, he may do best if allowed to choose the reward he will receive for completing work task prior to starting the work activity). Avoid rewards that are an "obsession" for him, such as small figurines and birds. Show him that after he works again, he gets the reward again. As the work is interspersed with rewards, gradually shape to include more work tasks between rewards.

7. If needed, use timer picture from Boardmaker or an auditory timer to indicate length of time he plays with the reward.
8. Once work activity routine is established, show the assistants how to implement the routine.

Teaching Plan for Objective 2

Objective 2: During structured play, Anthony will imitate adult play activities for 5 actions (actions with objects) with at least three different preferred objects (dinosaurs, animals, doll…) each day across 2 weeks.

Personal and Environmental Challenges and Supports for Teaching Plan 2

Personal challenges	*Environmental challenges*
• Lacks joint attention skills	• Is in an integrated setting with a lot of other students
• Lacks motivation to please others	• Physical distractions in the environment
• Lacks motivation for many objects/ activities	• Living arrangements at home have changed and are unstable
Personal supports	*Environmental supports*
• Likes animals and small animal toys he can hold in his hand	• Mother and teacher want same outcomes
• Has better receptive compared to expressive language skills	• Teacher and assistant know Anthony well
• Can imitate some actions with objects (drink from a cup)	• Has many social peers in his classroom
• Likes praise and hugs	• See teaching plan for specific supports and strategies to teach this skill

Teaching Plan

1. Refer to the Evidence-based Online Resources for Teachers in the forms section of Chap. 7, especially those on discrete trial training, prompting, and peer-mediated instruction.
2. Assemble objects that Anthony likes. Decide if you would like to use two identical objects so he can see what to do while simultaneously doing it or use one object with which to take turns.
3. Get Anthony's attention and imitate an action with the object (make a plane fly, a bear walk, a dog run, a rabbit hop, a car roll, etc.). Be creative and try out different things.
4. Give the object to Anthony and cue him "You do it" or a phrase you prefer to use to verbally cue him to perform the action with the object. If he has the same object, you might say, "Let's play, do this."
5. Use a system of least prompts and avoid physical assistance as much as possible. As long as he is watching, give him time to respond, otherwise cue him to look.

6. If he does the behavior, reward him with smiles, humming, and/or acknowledgment; if not, repeat from the second step.
7. If Anthony is taking turns imitating with one object, two objects are not needed.
8. Twirling and spinning things are highly preferred and interfering. They are not used to work on this skill, but might be used as reward if he understands when to give them up. Keep the toys that are allowed for spinning and reinforcement separate from those being used to teach appropriate use and imitation.
9. Generalize the verbal cues to include phrases paired with a gesture of holding a hand out to indicate "my turn."
10. Once the skill is mastered with one adult, generalize the skill to other adults and then begin to include a peer.

Teaching Plan for Objective 3

Objective 3: Anthony will make 10 different requests per day independently (go home, eat, help, more, finished, various objects/activities) or as a response to a question ("what do you want?") using sign, pictures, or verbalization on a daily basis across 2 weeks.

Personal and Environmental Challenges and Supports for Teaching Plan 3

Personal challenges	*Environmental challenges*
• Uses aggression to communicate many wants/needs/refusals, including confusion	• Is in an integrated setting with a lot of other students, making it difficult to provide intensive instruction
• Has low expressive language skills	• Has teaching assistants who are not trained
• Lacks motivation to please others	• Lacks consistency between home and school and use of visuals
• Lacks motivation for many objects/activities	
Personal supports	*Environmental support*
• Likes animals and small animal toys he can hold in his hand	• Has teacher who uses pictures/gestures to communicate
• Better receptive compared to expressive language skills	• Has access to pictures that can be used to express himself to others
• Understands many pictures	• Has mother and teacher who want same outcomes
	• Has teacher and assistant who know Anthony well
	• See teaching plan for specific supports and strategies

Teaching Plan

1. Refer to the Evidence-based Online Resources for Teachers in the forms section of Chap. 7, especially those on picture exchange communication system (PECS), functional communication training, and pivotal response training.

2. Begin to teach independent initiation; start with what he can currently do and expand. Begin with PECS. Also, implement naturalistic strategies based on functional communication training and pivotal response training.
3. Review with the teaching assistants the teaching methods of PECS online at: http://www.autisminternetmodules.org/mod_list.php.
4. Identify activities, objects, and other items that Anthony might like.
5. Develop a communication board with Boardmaker or photos that Anthony can pair with desires/needs.
6. Expand to other teaching situations to elicit requests, such as sabotaging a situation (e.g., place desired objects in view but out of reach or in a clear container with a tight lid). He really enjoys hand puppets. A clear container with a tight lid and a desired object inside can be used so that he has to ask for help.
7. Obtaining the object will be the reinforcer for Anthony to make the request.
8. Show you understand by complying with requests immediately and praising him.
9. Make sure that the team is clear on the method he needs to use to indicate the request (for instance, picture with verbalization or picture only). If he is not making requests independently or is being taught to request new items, he may need a second person who prompts him from behind when requesting with a picture.
10. Collaborate with the speech language pathologist in teaching this goal throughout the day and embed it within as many activities as possible. The more practice and success Anthony has, the quicker he will be able to learn this skill.

Summarize and Close

Next, the consultant distributed the COMPASS Consultation Satisfaction Questionnaire and COMPASS Fidelity Checklist to the parent and teacher. Because time was short, the consultant left the forms with the teacher and parent and asked that they be faxed when completed. The consultant also asked that an IEP meeting be arranged within the next 2 weeks so that the new objectives would be added. The first coaching session was scheduled.

Within a week of the consultation, a report of the consultation was sent via mail and email to the teacher and via mail to the parent. Enclosed with the report was information on dealing with sleeping and behavior problems. The parent-friendly resource materials came from the COMPASS series available online at www. ukautism.org. Also included in the report was a description of the teaching objectives, personal and environmental challenges and supports, and teaching plans.

The consultant made some observations of the parent, teacher, and teaching assistant following the consultation. Anthony's mother and teacher were quite involved during the discussion. They shared information and were active contributors; his teacher shared slightly more information than his mother. Both his teacher and mother appeared to benefit from additional insight into Anthony's needs and behavior. His mother, especially, needed more supports. There was much turmoil at home and Anthony, his mother, and siblings were living in temporary arrangements with the maternal grandmother due to a recent separation from Anthony's father. Thus, it was not clear how much Anthony's mother's interactions during the consultation were affected by stress from other problems and current living arrangements. When asked for possible replacement skills to teach, both his teacher and his parent needed assistance to generate ideas. Both his mother and teacher appeared extremely frustrated. When asked about the need for respite care at home, his mother became teary. The consultant solicited input directly by reviewing the information shared in the COMPASS Challenges and Supports Joint Summary Form and reminded them of the communication, social, and learning skills weaknesses that are being manifested as aggression. Anthony's teacher also appeared to be concerned about the number of children in her classroom overall and the number who had IEPs. The consultant reassured her that the teaching plans would be feasible and able to be implemented within the classroom. The teaching assistant was less involved, but reported how helpful the consultation was in helping her understand Anthony.

Coaching: Implementing Plans, Monitoring Progress, and Making Adjustments

Plan implementation and progress monitoring occurred throughout the year. As the plan was implemented, flexibility was encouraged for adjustments to be made readily and quickly as necessary depending on progress data. The four coaching sessions presented in this section took place about every 6 weeks. Coaching sessions can occur more frequently, but a minimum of four sessions is necessary. Recall that the coaching sessions are designed to facilitate teacher-implemented plans and procedures rather than consultant-implemented plans. A careful balance between consultant expertise in autism and teacher-directed teaching plans must be considered. As much as possible, the consultant encourages and supports ideas from the teacher using guided and Socratic questioning techniques discussed in Chap. 7. The implementation steps of the coaching sessions as described in Chap. 8 were followed (Table 9.3).

Coaching Session 1

During the first coaching session, much time was spent clarifying the teaching objectives and designing the teaching plans. To assist with these activities, the Session 1 Coaching Protocol provided in the forms section of Chap. 8 was followed. During the first coaching session, Ms. Caudill reported that the team was concerned

Table 9.3 Abridged COMPASS coaching protocol

See Chap. 8, Table 8.1 for full description of the procedural steps of the COMPASS Coaching Protocol

1. Observe the student demonstrating each targeted skill/objective/goal
2. Review the Goal Attainment Scale (GAS) Form
3. Complete the Teacher Interview for Coaching Form for each objective
4. Complete summary activities
5. Obtain completed evaluation and fidelity forms

about Anthony's level of aggression and that it might be unrealistic to expect him to meet the objective. The objective was slightly modified so that he was expected to start, but not complete, a task independently. It was clear that the teacher might have challenges in convincing her teaching assistants that Anthony could be successful beyond their expectations. This objective was added to the IEP. The consultant, however, with agreement from the teacher, retained the original objective developed during the consultation. The GAS Form based on the original objectives was reviewed with the teacher. Following this discussion, an observation of the instruction was conducted and also videotaped for each of the three targeted objectives for review with the teacher. Following the observation, the consultant and teacher met in a conference room and completed steps 3, 4, and 5 of the coaching protocol.

Step 1: Observe the Student Demonstrating Each Targeted Skill/Objective/Goal

The consultant and teacher observed videotape of Anthony and his teacher working on one of the three skills that were discussed during the consultation: "When presented with a task menu from which to select work tasks, Anthony will start and complete three 2–3 min tasks each day without aggression with one adult verbal cue (e.g., time to work) and gestural/picture cues across 2 weeks." We observed him completing a work task with multiple verbal and gestural cues from the teacher and no aggression. For the skill of learning to imitate play activities with at least three different preferred objects, opportunities to teach had not been created, according to Ms. Caudill. Therefore, we did not see a videotape of this skill. Instead, we observed this directly in the classroom. It was quite impressive to see Anthony sit down with Ms. Caudill, watch her imitate with an object, and then immediately imitate the same action with the object. He imitated at least two different objects. When given a toy dog, he was more focused on playing with the bird in a repetitive manner by flicking its wings repeatedly. But after some delay, Anthony was observed to imitate appropriate action with the toy dog. For the third skill, observation showed Anthony selecting a finished card and handing it to his teacher. More discussion about the skills follow.

Step 2: Review the Goal Attainment Scale Form

Goal attainment ratings were collected on the three primary skills. During the first coaching session, the GAS Form was introduced to Ms. Caudill and some of it was adjusted based on her input. For the first skill of "when presented with a task menu," a goal attainment score of −2 was observed. His teacher reported, however, that most of the time, Anthony was making progress and would fall at a −1 level.

For the second skill of "learning to imitate play activities with at least three different preferred objects," a GAS score of -1.5 was observed. His teacher, however, reported that most consistently he is scoring at a −2 level.

For the last skill of "initiating requests," a GAS score of −2 was observed. His teacher reported that Anthony consistently initiates about 2 to 3 requests daily independently.

Step 3: Complete the Teacher Interview Form for Each Objective

During the discussion with Ms. Caudill, the Teacher Interview for Coaching Form was completed. A copy of the form was provided to her to follow along. For the first skill of "when presented with a task menu," Ms. Caudill expressed concern that the objective appears to be two separate skills—to start an independent work task and to complete an independent work task. The consultant suggested that in the IEP, the skill may be broken down into two separate skills. For the consultation, however, it was preferred to keep them together as one skill because work completion was the primary aim, and starting a work task was the first step in learning to complete a work task independently. She agreed and reported that she worked on this skill on a daily basis. She also indicated that she was keeping data on this skill and needed no assistance with data collection (see the Activity-based Data Sheet below). She as well as the speech therapist both teach this skill. The speech therapist spent about 2 days a week in the classroom. Next, the teaching plan was reviewed. The teacher was mainly using a discrete trial approach and a lot of adult-directed prompting. Thus, the consultant reviewed the method of structured teaching as an alternative, evidence-based method that would support the development of independence. The consultant referred to the original consultation report that included online references, including video of structured teaching methods and ideas of developing further structured teaching types of activities.

Activity-Based Data Sheet

Student's Name: Anthony
Skill/Behavior: Start and complete work tasks.
Dates: Oct 5–16
Criterion Level: three 2–3 min work tasks with one adult verbal cue and gestural
            and visual cues
Coaching Session: 1
Prompt: (*circle*) I = Independent; V = Verbal; Vi = Visual; G = Gestural; P = Physical

Instructions: In the section above, describe the skill/behavior, criterion level,* and
circle the prompt(s) for the objective. Using the table below, list the prompts used,
tally the number of times the student demonstrated the skill at the criterion level
(# passed), and tally the number of opportunities provided (# opportunities). For the
bottom row, tally the total number of times passed and the total number of
opportunities.

Day		M	T	W	TH	F	M	T	W	TH	F
Date		10/5	10/6	10/7	10/8	10/9	10/12	10/13	10/14	10/15	10/16
Activities											
Independent work time in the morning	Prompt	5V	5V	5V	5V	5V	4V	4V	3V	3V	3V
		4P	4P	4P	4P	3P	3P	3P	2P	2P	1P
	# Passed	0	0	0	0	0	0	0	0	0	0
	# Opportunities	2	1	2	2	2	3	2	3	3	3
Speech and language therapy activities	Prompt		5V		5V			3V		3V	
			2P		2P			2P		2P	
	# Passed		0		0			0		0	
	# Opportunities		1		1			1		1	
Total	# Passed	0	0	0	0	0	0	0	0	0	0
	# Opportunities	2	2	2	3	2	3	3	3	4	3

*See Chap. 5 for more explanation on criterion level

For the second skill of "learning to imitate play activities with at least three
different preferred objects," Ms. Caudill reported that this was worked on once a
day. She said that she has seen him do this with two objects. The consultant saw this
during the observation as well as delayed imitation with the bird. The teacher was
not yet keeping data on the skill and has just recently started to work on it. She
indicated that she had a plan for data collection and did not need any assistance. She
also planned to use objects that were of less intense interest to Anthony to encourage more appropriate functional use of objects.

COMPASS Coaching Summary Template

Coaching Session (I)   II   III   IV

Student: ___anthony_____ Date:___September 23 School:__Sunshine El.___

Teacher: _Ms. Caudill_____ Consultant: __Ruble_____ OthersPresent:__None_____

Communication Skill: Initiating requests

Observation: We observed Anthony on tape selecting a finished card and handing it to his teacher.

Discussion: This skill has not been taught systematically. As a result, no data were being kept. His Teacher indicated that Anthony made about three to five requests a day and became upset about 75 percent of the time when he was denied a request. He used many symbols, such as a "help" symbol, a "more" symbol, a "finished" symbol, and a "go home" symbol about 50 percent of the time independently based on teacher report.

Goal Attainment: A goal attainment scale score of -2 was rated based on teacher report. His teacher reported that Anthony consistently initiates about 2 to 3 requests daily independently.

Social Skill: Imitating play

Observation: Opportunities to teach had not been created. We observed this skill directly in the classroom. It was quite impressive to see Anthony sit down with Ms. Caudill, watch her make actions with an object, and then immediately imitate the same action with the object. He imitated at least two different objects. When given a toy bird, he was more focused on playing with the bird in a repetitive manner by flicking its wings repeatedly. But after some delay, Anthony was observed to imitate appropriate action with the toy dog.

Discussion: This skill was worked on once a day. She said that she has seen him do this with two objects. The consultant saw this during the observation as well as delayed imitation with the bird. The teacher was not yet keeping data on the skill and has just recently started to work on it. She indicated that she had a plan for data collection and did not need any assistance. She also planned to use objects that were of less intense interest to Anthony to encourage more appropriate functional use of objects.

Goal Attainment: A goal attainment scale score of -1.5 was observed. His teacher, however, reported that most consistently he is scoring at a -2 level.

Learning Skill: starting and completing work tasks without aggression

Observation:. We observed him on tape completing a work task with multiple verbal and gestural cues from the teacher and no aggression.

Discussion: She as well as the speech therapist both teach this skill. The speech therapist spends about two days a week in the classroom. The teacher uses a discrete trial approach and a lot of adult-directed prompting. The method of structured teaching as an alternative, evidence-based method that would support the development of independence was suggested. The consultant referred to the original consultation report that included online references, including video of structured teaching methods and ideas of developing further structured teaching types of activities.

Goal Attainment: A goal attainment score of -2 was observed. His teacher reported, however, that most of the time, Anthony was making progress and would fall at a -1 level.

Future Plans:

1. Implement the teaching plans for all skills and be ready for us to observe or have a videotape.

2. Review the online resources of evidence based practice of structured teaching.

For the last skill of "initiating requests," she reported that this skill has not been taught systematically. As a result, no data were being kept. She indicated that Anthony made about three to five requests a day and became upset about 75% of the time when he was denied a request. He used many symbols, such as a "help" symbol, a "more" symbol, a "finished" symbol, and a "go home" symbol about 50% of the time independently.

Step 4: Complete Summary Activities

The consultation concluded with setting up the date and time of the next coaching session. The consultant also told the teacher that a summary report of the information collected and discussed during the coaching session (see example on page 215) would be provided within a week and sent to Anthony's teacher and parents (the Coaching Summary Template in Chap. 8 was used as a guide).

Step 5: Obtain Completed Evaluation and Fidelity Forms

Because so much information was shared with the teacher during the first coaching session, the consultant decided to delay collecting information from the teacher on her perceptions of coaching fidelity and satisfaction.

To obtain information on the overall impressions that the consultant had from the consultation and on the quality of teacher–student instruction, the consultant completed the Coaching Impressions Form (CIF), the Autism Engagement Rating Scale (AERS), and the Teacher Engagement Rating Scale (TERS). These forms are not necessary for COMPASS consultation, but may provide helpful qualitative information to consider for planning the next coaching section. The consultant judged the teacher as having implemented at least 75% of the teaching plans (a rating of 4- out of a 5-point scale) using the CIF item 10. The total rating of the quality of the child's engagement during the instruction using the AERS was 14 out of a total of 18 points, reflecting relatively high engagement. The teacher's quality of instruction using the TERS was rated 14.5 out of a total 18 points, reflecting relatively high engagement.

Coaching Session 2

All the steps completed in session one were completed in sessions two, three, and four using the Standard COMPASS Coaching Protocol in the forms section of Chap. 8. A brief description of each session is provided. Each description came from the coaching summary report that was written immediately following the consultation and mailed to the teacher and parent. Even though the parent was unable to attend the coaching sessions, she was mailed a copy of the summary.

Step 1: Observe the Student Demonstrating Each Targeted Skill/ Objective/Goal

The consultant observed Anthony and his teacher working on two of the three skills. The first skill was "when presented with a task menu, Anthony will start and complete three 2–3 min tasks each day." The consultant saw Anthony sorting quantities depicted on pictures. He worked up to four minutes easily. Verbal cuing was provided throughout.

For the second skill of "imitating adult play activities with at least three different preferred objects," the consultant observed Anthony and his teacher taking turns with a dog puppet. Anthony was smiling, following Ms. Caudill's directions of what to do with the object and readily taking turns with the object by handing it back to Ms. Caudill when she used a verbal and gestural (hand extended outward) cue.

For the last skill of "making ten different requests per day independently," the consultant did not observe the skill. But Ms. Caudill reported that he does request "more," "help," "bathroom," "home," "eat," and "finish" spontaneously.

Step 2: Review the Goal Attainment Scale Form

Goal attainment ratings were collected. For the first skill of "when presented with a task menu from which to select a work task," a goal attainment score of +2 was observed and also reported by his teacher. Anthony was working at least four minutes at a time and this was to be expanded to be done with other adults.

For the second skill of "imitating adult play activities," a GAS score of +2 was observed and also reported by his teacher. This skill was to be expanded to be done with other adults, peers, or in small group settings.

For the last skill of "making requests," a score of −1 for making progress was reported but not observed. Clearly, Anthony was making significant and meaningful progress.

Step 3: Complete the Teacher Interview Form for Each Objective

During the discussion with Ms. Caudill, the consultant reviewed each skill and asked the same questions covered during the first coaching session: how many times a day or week the skill was worked on, whether data were being collected, who taught the skill, and any other issues that needed to be addressed. The consultant also referred to the coaching summary report from the last session, the GAS Form, and the teaching plans for each skill. The teaching plan for each skill was updated, if necessary, to make sure it was reflecting the current strategies.

For the first skill, "when presented with a task menu," Ms. Caudill reported that this skill continues to be worked on a daily basis, about three to four times a day. She was collecting data and agreed to provide data on his progress within the week. She reported that both she and the teaching assistant worked on this skill. Anthony tended to be more responsive to Ms. Caudill's instruction compared to the instruction coming from the assistant. Ms. Caudill thought it would be good for Anthony to learn to accept instruction from others and said she would start working on this. The consultant also talked about this skill as written on the GAS Form, including both starting and finishing a task. Although the IEP only asks about starting a task, the teacher was collecting data on both starting and finishing. The consultant discussed online training resources and referred the teacher to those on structured teaching. Overall, the consultant was extremely impressed with how well Anthony was doing with this objective. He was working four to five minutes at a time with no aggression.

For the second skill of "learning to imitate adult play activities with at least three different preferred objects," Ms. Caudill reported that this was worked on twice a day. She said that Anthony imitated many objects, but that she avoided objects of strong interest (like birds or objects with wings). It was fantastic to see Anthony laughing and enjoying "playing" and imitating Ms. Caudill during the observation. She also built in additional concepts such as taking turns and identifying body parts in the interaction. The consultant talked about expanding his imitation interactions to other people and even peers. She is keeping data on the skill using the Activity-Based Data Sheet.

For the last skill of "making ten different requests daily," the consultant discussed the various requests Anthony makes independently. He asked for "more," "toilet," "home," "eat," "help," and "finish." He requested help about three to four times a day. We talked about setting up situations to sabotage, and Ms. Caudill has many ideas about this to try out. With the speech therapist, she worked on making requests using a second person behind Anthony to cue him to the conversational partner.

Activity-Based Data Sheet

Student's Name: Anthony
Skill/Behavior: During structured play will imitate adult play (actions with
                objects)
Dates: Dec 7–18
Criterion Level: Five actions with three different preferred objects
Coaching Session: 2
Prompt: (*circle*) I = Independent; V = Verbal; Vi = Visual; G = Gestural; P = Physical

Day		M	T	W	TH	F	M	T	W	TH	F
Date		12/7	12/8	12/9	12/10	12/11	12/14	12/15	12/16	12/17	12/18
Activities											
Morning free play	Prompt	1V	1V	1V	1V	1V	1V	1V	1V	1V	1V
	#Passed	2	2	2	2	3	3	1	3	3	3
	#Opportunities	3	3	3	3	3	3	3	3	3	3
Circle time	Prompt	2V	2V	1V	1V	1V	1V	1V	1V	1V	1V
	#Passed	0	0	1	1	3	3	3	3	3	3
	#Opportunities	3	3	3	3	3	3	3	3	3	3
Total	#Passed	2	2	3	3	6	6	4	6	5	6
	#Opportunities	6	6	6	6	6	6	6	6	6	6

Step 4: Complete Summary Activities

The consultant reminded Ms. Caudill to fax the data sheets within the week. The date for the next session was set, and a report was written and sent within the week.

Step 5: Obtain Completed Evaluation and Fidelity Forms

Ms. Caudill completed the Coaching Feedback Form (see Chap. 8). Her ratings indicated that the coaching sessions had been generally well received. She gave a mean rating of 3.25 out of 4 for the 4 coaching session items, and a mean rating of 3 out of 4 for the four consultant items. She indicated that the discussions were most helpful.

Coaching Session 3

Step 1: Observe the Student Demonstrating Each Targeted Skill/ Objective/Goal

For the first skill of "starting and completing a work task," the consultant observed Anthony working one-on-one with Ms. Caudill on a number of identification tasks. He appeared to be growing frustrated (demonstrated by not responding or tossing the object) with the tasks. From the consultant's perspective, possible reasons appeared to be because he wanted a different reward or because he wanted to be done with the task. Ms. Caudill interpreted that he wanted a different motivator, and she went to a container with various toys and brought it back to the table for Anthony to see. This immediately perked Anthony up, and he completed the tasks with no further objection. She remained calm and persistent with him to complete the task despite his initial frustration and lack of desire to finish. Anthony expressed frustration in a nonaggressive way, and it was clear to the consultant that he had made a lot of progress in this area.

For the next skill of "imitating adult play activities," the consultant observed Anthony playing a role in a skit about Brown Bear. He took a turn in the role of Brown Bear and was cued to hold a large cutout of a circle in front of his face. He responded well, was a part of the group, and was doing what the other children were doing.

For the last skill of "making 10 different requests," no observation was done, but Ms. Caudill reported that he was making at least 10–15 requests per day. She also indicated that lunch time would be a good time to capture him making several requests.

Step 2: Review the Goal Attainment Scale Form

Using the GAS Form, Ms. Caudill reported that Anthony was at the expected level of outcome for the first skill of initiating and completing a task and received a GAS score of 0. The consultant also observed this during the video.

For the second skill of imitating adult play activities, Anthony exceeded expectations and was at the +1 level. This was reported by Ms. Caudill as his most consistent level of performance. It was also observed by the consultant. Anthony was generalizing his skills from adults to children.

For the last skill of "making 10 different requests," his teacher reported that he is between the 0 and +1, a GAS score of +0.5. Unfortunately, the consultant was not able to observe this that day.

Step 3: Complete the Teacher Interview for Coaching Form for Each Objective

For the first skill of "starting and completing a task," Ms. Caudill reported that this was worked on at least four times a day. She kept data on this skill as well as the other skills. She said that he still had difficulty with some of the teaching assistants. She said she wanted to work on generalizing his abilities to work with other adults besides herself. She said she would start to have Anthony complete work tasks in the new classroom to facilitate his transition into Kindergarten.

For the next skill of "imitating adult actions," Ms. Caudill reported she was working on this about twice per day. She said that recently she saw Anthony imitating the other peers washing dishes without any adult modeling. This was an excellent sign, as his awareness had grown so much and his imitation skills were expanding from not just imitating adult actions but peer actions as well. Anthony also imitated stacking blocks and movements with small animals. His teacher had made videotapes to depict the positive skill of taking turns and imitating peer models for Anthony to view. Ms. Caudill had a plan of showing him this for a few days in a row and then having him do the behavior shown on the tape with a peer.

For the last skill of "making 10 different requests per day," Ms. Caudill reported that Anthony was making 10–15 requests per day (see activity based data sheet).

Activity-Based Data Sheet

Student's Name: Anthony
Skill/Behavior: make requests or respond to "what do you want" using sign, pictures, or vocalizations

Dates: March 3–14
Criterion Level: Ten per day independently
Coaching Session: 4
Prompt: (circle) I=Independent V = Verbal; Vi = Visual; G = Gestural; P = Physical

Day		M	T	W	TH	F	M	T	W	TH	F
Date		3/3	3/4	3/5	3/6	3/7	3/10	3/11	3/12	3/13	3/14
Activities											
Breakfast	Prompt	1	1	1V	1V	1V	1	1	1	1	1
		V/P	V/P								
	# Passed	3	3	3	3	3	3	3	2	3	2
	# Opportunities	3	3	3	3	3	3	3	2	3	2
Speech language therapy	Prompt	V	V	V	V	1	1	1	1	1	1
	# Passed	5	5	7	8	10	10	10	10	10	10
	# Opportunities	10	10	10	10	10	10	10	10	10	10
Sabotaged situations during work time	Prompt	1	1	1							
		V/P	V/P	V/P							
	# Passed	0	0	0							
	# Opportunities	2	2	2							
Total	# Passed	7	7	9	11	13	13	13	12	13	12
	# Opportunities	12	12	12	13	13	13	13	12	13	12

Step 4: Complete Summary Activities

The next coaching session was scheduled. Included in the summary was praise for the teacher on how much progress Anthony has made.

Step 5: Obtain Completed Evaluation and Fidelity Forms

The consultant asked the teacher to complete the Coaching Feedback Form, but it was not returned. It was decided that the additional forms would be distributed every other session at most.

Coaching Session 4

Step 1: Observe the Student Demonstrating each Targeted Skill/ Objective/Goal

For the first skill of "starting and completing 2–3 min tasks," the consultant observed Anthony trying to be redirected by his teacher to the work task while he was asking for a dinosaur. Ms. Caudill reported that although aggression was not observed, aggression had increased in the last several weeks. Nevertheless, when he was requesting dinosaurs and told "no," he was not observed to hit or slap like he did at the beginning of the year.

For the second skill of "imitating adult play activities," the consultant observed several video clips of Anthony involved with peer activities. Taping these skills for viewing by the consultant at a later time was easier for the teacher because she was able to capture naturalistic interactions and instruction that occurred during regular classroom routines (rather than setting up a situation when the consultant was there). In one clip, Anthony was sitting on the floor with a baby doll and other toys. Two children playing with facemasks were sitting next to him. There was not a lot of interaction between the two other children and Anthony, but it was clear that the children were comfortable being around Anthony, and Anthony was showing more awareness of the other children. In the second video clip, Anthony was sitting on a chair next to the sandbox where all of the children were playing. He was taking the sand and letting it fall between his fingers and watching the other children.

For the last skill of "making ten different requests," we saw Anthony using signs, pictures, and words. There were several situations observed where he used a picture to indicate help.

Step 2: Review the Goal Attainment Scale Form

For the first skill of "starting and completing a work task without aggression," Ms. Caudill reported that Anthony was at the −1.5 level. We also observed this during the observation.

For the second skill of "imitating adult play activities," Ms. Caudill reported that Anthony was at the +1 level. He was doing much more imitation play with other children. The consultant observed this and also scored him at a +1 level.

For the last skill of "making at least ten different requests," Anthony's teacher reported that he was at the 0 level most consistently. The consultant also observed him performing at this level.

Step 3: Complete the Teacher Interview for Coaching Form for each objective

For the first skill of "starting and completing a work task," Ms. Caudill reported that starting without any aggression had been difficult recently and that Anthony had regressed; however, once he started the work, Anthony completed tasks without aggression. According to this teacher, spring break occurred a couple weeks before this consultation, and Anthony usually required more time to settle into his routines after breaks. The consultant reminded the teacher that school absences and holiday breaks are an environmental challenge for Anthony, and that environmental supports needed to be enhanced to overcome the challenges. One support for Anthony following breaks was use of established routines rather than the introduction of new activities. Ms. Caudill was working with his teaching assistants so that Anthony would become more accepting of different people working with him during his activities. Ms. Caudill reported that this skill was worked on about seven times a day.

The consultant reviewed the teaching plan. Ms. Caudill was still working with all of the strategies listed on the plan. The only one she was not using was a mini schedule. The consultant suggested that a picture of the work activity and a picture of the reward be shown to Anthony. The consultant also suggested having Ms. Caudill be the one who works with him primarily for a few days after breaks so that established routines were used until he became stable. It was then suggested that changes be planned to happen one at a time, so that the assistant would work with him after his aggression was reduced. Also discussed was the possibility of Ms. Caudill taping the assistant working with Anthony and also the teacher working with Anthony. The teacher could then show these tapes to the assistant so she could become more aware of how she was instructing and more aware of her use of the word "no," which was a personal challenge for Anthony.

For the next skill of "imitating adult play activities," Ms. Caudill reported that this was worked on about ten times per day. She said that overall Anthony had engaged in many spontaneous peer interactions and was participating in circle time. The consultant saw a video clip of circle time, and the teacher also kept data on this skill. The consultant reviewed the teaching strategies and the only strategy added was to discuss with the peers individually how to get Anthony's attention, keep Anthony's attention, and play with Anthony. The consultant provided some suggestions and a script that could be used for the peer training. The teacher reported that there were two to three girls who had enjoyed being a peer coach for Anthony. The teacher agreed that she, the speech language pathologist, and peers would work on this skill with Anthony.

For the last skill of "making 10 different requests per day independently," the teacher reported that breakfast was an opportunity that was often used to make several requests. Such requests included not only asking for food but also requesting help. The teacher as well as the speech language therapist and assistants worked with Anthony on this skill approximately 12 times a day. The teaching plan was also reviewed. The consultant found that all the strategies were being used except for the use of a very tight container with a desired object inside. The teacher reported that this made him very upset and that she did not want to continue with this strategy. A copy of his Activity-based Data Sheet is provided (see next page).

Step 4: Complete Summary Activities

The consultant acknowledged with the teacher how much progress Anthony made throughout the year. The GAS Form was reviewed and current scores were compared to scores from the beginning of the year. At the start of the year, Anthony was unable to complete any of the tasks. He made significant progress on all skills, with the exception of starting a work task without aggression. He appeared to regress after break, and the need for more supports was necessary. Over the year, numerous environmental supports were put into place for Anthony.

These supports were not removed given how much he needed consistency. The consultant reviewed these environmental supports with Ms. Caudill, who planned to facilitate his transition into kindergarten and to help ensure these supports were in place.

Step 5: Obtain Completed Evaluation and Fidelity Forms

Ms. Caudill completed the COMPASS Coaching Fidelity Checklist. A mean rating of 3.4 out of 4 for the 19 items was calculated, indicating that the consultant followed the procedures of the COMPASS Coaching Protocol with adequate fidelity from the teacher's perspective. The consultant also completed the COMPASS Coaching Impressions Scale. The teacher received an overall rating of 4 out of 5 points for adherence to the teaching plans (item 10 on the form). Thus, overall the teacher implemented most of the teaching plans as written.

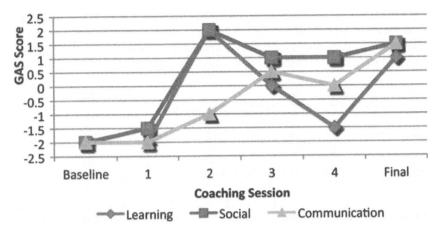

Fig. 9.1 Anthony's GAS scores by coaching session

Final Evaluation of Progress

Figure 9.1 shows Anthony's progress using the GAS Form and the overall mean scores by coaching session. Progress was made for all skills, but progress was also sporadic. Most difficult for Anthony was the number of holiday breaks and snow days. Coaching sessions 3 and 4 demonstrated evidence of the drop in progress following days away from school. Nevertheless, Anthony did achieve all his skills at levels that exceeded expectations.

Case Study 2: Ethan

Background Information

Ethan was an 8-year-old Caucasian boy who attended an elementary school in a rural area located in a southern state. Ethan spent most of his academic time in a special education classroom, but he did participate with children in the general education setting for some academic work and for art, recess, and physical education. He received speech, language, and occupational therapy at school. At the start of the consultation, Ethan had been receiving about 10 h a week of applied behavior analysis therapy at home for the previous 2 years.

Ethan lived with his parents and toddler sister and preschool brother in a new home that they just moved into when the school year started. His mother worked part-time. His mother and father were highly committed and involved with Ethan. One parent attended all teacher coaching sessions following the initial COMPASS consultation.

His teacher was very interested in learning all she could about autism and meeting the needs of not only Ethan, but other students with ASD whom she taught. She was selected by her school system to be a member of a training team on ASD being conducted by her state's Department of Education.

Step A: Activities Prior to COMPASS Consultation

Step A. 1. Gather Information About the Student from Consultant Observations and from Parent and Teacher Report Using the COMPASS Challenges and Supports Form for Caregivers and Teachers

When the consultation began, Ethan's IEP stated that he demonstrated the ability to understand almost everything that was said to him. He used words and phrases to communicate, and although he had spontaneous speech, he more often than not repeated what he had heard. He had great trouble with conversational speech. Ethan also required numerous prompts to complete tasks. He counted by rote, recognized letters, and demonstrated that he knew most letter sounds. Ethan did not do well in unstructured time and got off task frequently. Ethan had low muscle tone. Socially, Ethan was more comfortable with adults than peers. He typically engaged in parallel play and imitated motions of peers. He was developing some problem-solving skills.

Information from direct evaluation: The consultant conducted a standardized assessment of Ethan's cognitive, language, adaptive, and behavior skills. Ethan received a standard score of 63 for cognitive and problem-solving skills based on the Differential Abilities Scale. This score was significantly below average. He received a standard score of 41 for listening and verbal skills on the Oral and Written Language Scales, and a standard score of 64 for adaptive behavior skills based on teacher report using the Vineland Adaptive Behavior Scale. His teacher completed the Behavioral Assessment Scale for children, and a T score of 57 was calculated for externalizing behaviors, indicating no significant behavioral concerns. Lastly, a score of 33 was determined using the Childhood Autism Rating Scale, indicating mild/moderate autism.

Step A. 2. Complete COMPASS Challenges and Supports Joint Summary Form

Before the consultation began, Ethan's parents and his teachers—both general education and special education teachers together—completed the COMPASS Challenges and Supports Form for Caregivers and Teachers. The consultant then summarized their responses using the joint summary form.

Step B. Activities during a COMPASS Consultation

Step B. 1. Discuss COMPASS Consultation Training Packet

The consultation was held in the conference room at the school with Ethan's teacher, Ms. Hardin, and his mother, Ms. Jacobs. There seemed to be good rapport between the teacher and the parent as they shared information freely about personal events. All the information in the COMPASS Consultation Training Packet was discussed, including the purpose of the consultation, best practices, resources, and the iceberg illustration. Then the consultation quickly centered on Ethan. After the consultation, Ethan's mother commented to the consultant how helpful the session had been and that she hoped it would help with follow-through.

Step B. 2. Discuss COMPASS Consultation Joint Summary

A review of Ethan's likes and preferences began the discussion. Ethan enjoyed swimming, swinging, music and playing the piano, horseback riding, writing numbers and letters, shopping, eating at restaurants, playing in the resistance tunnel at school, repeating what annoyed someone over and over, all kinds of movement, riding on the bus, Clifford, Walmart, basketball, riding the scooter, candy corn, marshmallows, and raisins.

His parents listed Ethan's strengths and abilities as being very happy and always smiling, making tremendous progress, enjoying being with people, teasing and being very playful, and being full of life with unlimited potential. His teachers wrote that once he had learned something, he had it; he learned routines and schedules quickly, was willing to try new things, was able to communicate wants and needs effectively, and was very likeable and very observant.

His teachers and parents had high agreement about Ethan's personal challenges. In the area of personal management, these included waiting, being quiet when required, listening, accepting "no," staying where he was supposed to stay, changing activities at school, and going places in the community.

His fears and frustrations were listed as dogs, hospitals and doctor's offices, Lowes and other places with high ceilings, loud and sudden noises, being physically restrained, being in confined spaces, and having to participate in required activities such as tornado drills. Ethan wanted to interact appropriately with peers, and he became frustrated when he was unable to do so. He liked to be in control and became upset when things changed. Not getting what he wanted and having to sit still and be quiet was frustrating for Ethan.

Communication concerns included not asking for help at school and instead demanding "I want _____." At home, he talked repeatedly about past events and expressed anxiety by indicating he did not want something by adding "No" in front of the word (e.g., "No store today"). When he was confused at school, he made whining noises and said "I want _____." Sometimes when he became angry, mad, or frustrated, he escalated to pinching or pulling hair and saying, "Daddy says..." or "I want Daddy." Also he sometimes said, "I want time out."

Ethan showed his strongest social abilities at home with adults—his parents. They were the most predictable people for him. With his parents, he reportedly initiated social interactions, pointed at an object to direct their attention to share enjoyment, used greetings spontaneously (with children at home too), and took turns within familiar routines. At home, he also played games that were repetitive, imitated and expanded on actions with objects, and responded to another person's approach by smiling or vocalizing (he also did this at school with adults). His strength with children at home, school, and other places was accepting them being close to him; he could also imitate what another person did with an object in a variety of contexts. He imitated sounds and body movements. He generally looked where a person was pointing, with the exception at home with children. Ethan was not able to maintain social interactions or consistently respond to or initiate interactions with others.

Ethan had numerous sensory-related events that were problems for him. He reacted to unexpected sounds, feared some noises, was distracted by noises, and made self-induced noises. He had trouble masking out sound and listening to what was said to him at school. At school, he was reported to be very distracted by sounds and noises. He sought out the microwave and mini-processor. Ethan had trouble with eye contact and following with his eyes. He enjoyed watching bright, moving objects and liked the computer.

At school, it was reported that he disliked having his eyes covered and could see objects far away. There were no concerns noted in the olfactory area. In the tactile area, it was reported that Ethan liked deep touching and hugs when he initiated them. He disliked the feel of certain clothing and at school refused to touch some gooey things. Ethan liked water and mouthed some things. He preferred being barefooted; at home, he liked rough and tumble play and being wrapped up, but he did not like to be physically restrained. He liked to touch necks, but he did not like to touch using the very tips of his fingers.

For taste, he has definite preferences in foods, and at school they reported that he disliked certain foods and textures and that he tasted and that he mouthed nonedibles. Ethan liked to run and move. He liked spinning, rocking, swinging, and bouncing. He paced the floor at home when nervous. His teachers reported he climbed and bumped into things and people. Ethan also had trouble with paper/pencil activities at school, using some tools, and was very distracted by things moving around him.

As the team reviewed the information in the COMPASS Challenges and Supports Joint Summary Form, the consultant clarified and made sure that everyone had a solid understanding of Ethan within the context of the COMPASS Model. The consultant emphasized it was necessary for all participants to understand Ethan's personal challenges and environmental challenges so the team could work together to balance these with the personalized and needed supports. The team needed to know about Ethan's personal supports in order to move forward to address the environmental supports/teaching plans to help him continue to make progress and be a competent learner. That his involved parents and his teachers worked together certainly was an environmental support for Ethan.

The consultant explained that Ethan's frustration and agitation—as evidenced by his repeated talking, which if unchecked often escalated into a whine and eventually led to misbehavior—was like the tip of the iceberg. Below the surface were his fears, frustrations, and concerns. When these underlying issues were not addressed adequately, Ethan's negative behavior could escalate and he was not able to process his parents' or teachers' explanations or reasoning.

Step B. 3. Identify and Come to Consensus on Three Prioritized Objectives and Write Measurable Objectives

Following the discussion of the joint summary forms, the team discussed what three skills to target for coaching throughout the year. The consultant reminded the team to address skills that represented each of the core areas of autism—communication and social skills. These were both skill areas his parents and teachers felt needed to be addressed. The other area that emerged from much discussion was his ability to self-regulate or stay calm when confronted with his various frustrations and fears.

The agreed-upon objectives were as follows:

1. Communication: Ethan will give full-sentence answers when asked about his specific past experiences that day for three exchanges on three topics a day for 5 consecutive days.
2. Social/Communication: During a 10-min structured play activity with a peer, Ethan will make five appropriate comments. He will be able to do this during five consecutive activities during 1 week.
3. Personal Management/Adaptive Skills: Ethan will follow a relaxation routine with two verbal cues and visual cues and be able to continue in the current activity or setting without escalating behaviors (whining, yelling out) on five consecutive occasions when he is starting to be upset/anxious.

Step B. 4. Develop COMPASS Teaching Plans for Each Measurable Objective

The teaching plans for each objective were written together during this consultation session with the knowledge that the objectives would be added to Ethan's IEP before the first coaching session and that the teaching plans would be reviewed and updated at each coaching session. The plans were viewed as a work in progress that the team approached collaboratively. Resources and examples were provided so the teacher felt competent in implementing the agreed-upon plans.

Teaching Plan for Objective 1

Objective 1: Ethan will give full-sentence answers when asked about his specific past experiences that day for three exchanges on three topics a day for five consecutive days.

Personal and Environmental Challenges and Supports for Teaching Plan 1

Personal challenges	Environmental challenges
• Usually answers in one-word sentences	• Is distracted by noises and objects in the environment
• Lacks spontaneous commenting	
• Is unable to converse back and forth	
• Lacks the words to say what he did	
Personal supports	Environmental supports
• Does a variety of activities	• Has family that works to generalize and use skills
• Is beginning to read	• See teaching plan for specific supports and strategies to teach this skill
• Likes numbers	

Teaching Plan

1. Refer to the Online Resources for Teachers in the forms section of Chap. 7, in particular the resources on communication interventions.
2. Develop conversational scripts that interest Ethan and that he can use to communicate about his day.
3. Expand scripts to home and school.
4. Develop a list of questions that he can be asked at home (about school) and at school (about home).
5. Develop a schedule of his daily and weekly activities to share with home that can be used to ask questions.

    (a) Script might be "Did you like art today (or what did you do in art or other activities today)?"
    (b) Scripts might include choices for Ethan to check off when answering the conversational partner.

    For example,

    i. "I did like art."
    ii. "I did not like art today."

6. When he returns from the first grade, engage Ethan in a routine commenting about what he did to one of the assistants or his teacher. Let him know that he

will do this with Grandma, Mom, and Dad too. Also, practice with adults in the classroom before he leaves for the day.
7. Reinforce him with your enjoyment in sharing with him.

Teaching Plan for Objective 2

Objective 2: During a 10-min structured play activity with a peer, Ethan will make five appropriate comments. He will be able to do this during five consecutive activities during 1 week.

Personal and Environmental Challenges and Supports for Teaching Plan 2

Personal challenges	*Environmental challenges*
• Seldom comments with peers now	• Is distracted by environmental noises and objects
• Often makes a one-word comment or uses a learned script now when commenting	• Has few sociable peers who will stick with him and learn a script
• Watches peers more than being engaged with them	
Personal supports	*Environmental supports*
• Likes kids and watches them	• Has parent and teacher who communicate regularly with each other
• Seems to want to participate but doesn't know how	• See teaching plan for specific supports and strategies to teach this skill
• Has similar interests to his peers	
• Has good physical skills and interests such as basketball	

Teaching Plan

1. Review to the Online Resources for Teachers in the forms section of Chap. 7, especially those on video modeling, social narrative, social interventions, peer-mediated instructions and interventions, and communication.
2. Select activities and peers who can participate on a regular basis.
3. Use a social story that includes talking to friends and the things they like to talk about.
4. Plan a script to teach the peer and Ethan.
5. Use visual cue cards with comments and teach Ethan to read the comment cards.
6. Demonstrate through a video tape or in real time video that demonstrates Ethan and the other children commenting during play.
7. Start with activities and a time frame that is comfortable for Ethan, then add to activities.

Teaching Plan for Objective 3

Objective 3: Ethan will follow a relaxation routine with two verbal cues and visual cues and be able to continue in the current activity or setting without escalating behaviors (whining, yelling out) on five consecutive occasions when he is starting to be upset/anxious.

Personal and Environmental Challenges and Supports for Teaching Plan 3

Personal challenges	Environmental challenges
• Has anxiety about a number of things, i.e. being told no, being corrected, needing help, dogs, doctor's offices, being held down in tornado drill, Walmart, some areas with high ceilings, not understanding, being confused, changes in schedules, some elevators, not being able to do what he wants at times (run, use the microwave at home)	• Has trouble to responding to directions given from others at school and home, especially at school • Has difficulty with changes that occur at school and home • Has to encounter dogs and other things that might bother him
Personal supports	
• Likes routines and easily learns to follow them • Imitates well • Responds to scripts and learns quickly • Likes to count • Is familiar with "count and blow"	• His parents who also work on this skill and continue to challenge him to expand his interests and address his fears • See teaching plan for specific supports and strategies to teach this skill

Teaching Plan

1. Review to the Online Resources for Teachers in the forms section of Chap. 7, especially those on social narratives, video modeling, differential reinforcement, relaxation/calming, and self-management.
2. Write a social story with Ethan about calming down.
3. Develop a routine that is based on his interests and strengths (counting and blowing) that is practiced daily.
4. Teach him to respond to the verbal cue "Calm down Ethan and count" and the visual cue (numbers that increase from 1 to 10) and include an adult model demonstrating the skill as he imitates that adult.
5. Practice the routine using the same cues (verbal and picture) several times a day in various settings when Ethan is calm.
6. Anytime Ethan starts to whine, use the calm down routine.

7. Develop a visual cue card or several cards that Ethan can carry with him and use during the routine. Later, this can become his cue card rather than the adult verbal cues.
8. Try taping Ethan using the calm down routine and showing the tape to him.
9. Consider whether a self-monitoring system might be used to remind him to stay calm and what to do if he needs to calm down.

Goal Attainment Scale Form for Ethan

−2 Present level of performance	−1 Progress	0 Expected level of outcome (GOAL)	+1 Somewhat more than expected	+2 Much more than expected
Usually answers in one-word sentences. Not much spontaneous commenting or back-and-forth conversation. Doesn't have the words to say what he did in the past	Ethan shall give full-sentence answers when asked about his specific past experiences that day for 3 (1–2) exchange on 3 (1–2) topics a day for 5 (2) consecutive days	Ethan shall give full-sentence answers when asked about his specific past experiences that day for 3 exchanges on 3 topics a day for 5 consecutive days	Ethan shall give full-sentence answers independently when asked about his past experiences that day for 3 (4) exchanges on 3 (4) topics a day for 5 (7) consecutive days (with peers)	Ethan shall give full-sentence answers independently when asked about his specific past experiences that day for 3 (6) exchanges on 3 (6) topics a day for 5 (10) consecutive days (with peers)
Seldom comments with peers. Often makes a one-word comment or learned script. Watches peers more than is engaged with them	During a structured play activity with a peer, Ethan shall make 5 (2) appropriate comments. He will be able to do this during 5 (2) consecutive activities during 1 week	During a structured play activity with a peer, Ethan shall make 5 appropriate comments. He will be able to do this during 5 activities during 1 week	During a structured play activity with a peer, Ethan shall make 5 (7) appropriate comments. He will be able to do this during 5 (7) consecutive activities during 1 week	During a structured play activity with a peer, Ethan shall make 5 (10) appropriate comments. He will be able to do this during 5 (10) consecutive activities during 1 week

(continued)

(continued)

−2 Present level of performance	−1 Progress	0 Expected level of outcome (GOAL)	+1 Somewhat more than expected	+2 Much more than expected
Anxious about many things (being told no, being corrected, needing help, dogs, doctors' offices, being held down in tornado drill, Walmart, some areas with high ceilings, changes in schedules, some elevators, not being able to do what he wants. Paces, hums, or says he wants to go home when upset. Does not use words to express when upset/anxious	Ethan shall follow a relaxation routine with 2 (3+) verbal cues and visual cues and be able to continue in the current activity or setting without escalating behaviors (whining, yelling out) on 5 (2) consecutive occasions when he is starting to be upset/anxious	Ethan shall follow a relaxation routine with 2 verbal cues and visual cues and be able to continue in the current activity or setting without escalating behaviors (whining, yelling out) on 5 consecutive occasions when he is starting to be upset/anxious	Ethan shall follow a relaxation routine with 2 (1) verbal cues and visual cues and be able to continue in the current activity or setting without escalating behaviors (whining, yelling out) on 5 (7) consecutive occasions when he is starting to be upset/anxious	Ethan shall follow a relaxation routine with 2 (0) verbal cues and visual cues and be able to continue in the current activity or setting without escalating behaviors (whining, yelling out) on 5 (10) consecutive occasions when he is starting to be upset / anxious

Coaching Session 1

The session occurred 1 month following the consultation at Ethan's school in the conference room with his teacher and mother present. His teacher provided an updated IEP with the new objectives included. The consultant and his mother viewed a videotape clip of Ethan performing each skill. Following each clip, a discussion took place using the Teacher Interview for Coaching Form. Efficient ways to keep data on each skill were also discussed. The GAS Form (see previous page) was reviewed with input from everyone, and Ethan's performance at school and at home was rated.

Communication Skills

For the communication objective of using complete sentences in answer to questions, Ms. Hardin had begun to use a task-analysis approach. The consultant observed her scripting the conversation for Ethan with fill-in-the-blank responses.

He read the sentence and wrote the appropriate response. He then referred to the written script to provide full-sentence answers to questions. He required several verbal and gestural cues to complete the task. Ms. Hardin is working on this skill with Ethan about four times a week. Mrs. Hardin sent the scripted paper home with Ethan so that he and his parents could practice at home and so that his parents were informed about what Ethan did at school. Ethan also had a home script that was completed and returned to school so that he could answer questions from his teacher about home. The team discussed whether or not the inclusion of visual supports be listed in his objective, and it was agreed that the expected level of outcome should include the use of visual supports to facilitate independence (no adult verbal cuing). Ethan's mother reported that he was using complete sentences more frequently with her. He received a GAS score of −1.

Social Skills

For the social/communication objective of making appropriate comments during structured play, this skill was just beginning to be worked on and was instructed four times a week. The team brainstormed activities that would hold Ethan's interest and for which peers might be supportive. He received a GAS score of -1.5.

Personal Management/Adaptive Skills

On the personal management objective of following a relaxation routine, Ethan's mother said that she had been experimenting with a routine at home and found that he did best using a card with numbers 1–10 on it as a reminder and then the verbal cues and model of "count and blow." It was agreed that because he could and would do this routine it would be used everywhere with the cue, "Ethan, count and blow." He received a GAS score of −1.5.

Summary Activities

The time for the next coaching session was set for about 3 weeks after the winter holiday break. A summary of the coaching session was then sent to Ethan's teacher and his parents within a week. The GAS Form and changes in the teaching plan were included with the summary of the discussion.

Coaching Session 2

The second coaching session was held about 5 weeks after the first. Ethan's father and teacher were present. Since the first coaching session, there had been 2 weeks of holiday break and several snow days. In spite of these interruptions, Ethan continued to make progress. As before, the team reviewed the skills by observing Ethan via videotape.

Communication Skills

On the communication objective of responding in full sentences, Ethan's teaching assistant was observed working with him on this skill during the instruction to help generalize his skills across people. Ethan answered questions readily using the script. His answers appeared well rehearsed and almost rote. It was not clear if he was listening to the question or what he might have done if a different question was asked. The objective was being worked on daily and data were being kept. The team discussed fading out some of the visual cues to encourage and challenge Ethan to think through his answers and listen more carefully to the questions. The consultant also talked about the need for his parents to share more information so that Ethan could better answer questions at school about home. His father said that Ethan was constantly asking to go to Walmart, and the consultant and teacher suggested putting Walmart on the calendar so that Ethan had a visual reference. He received a GAS score of 0.

Social Skills

On the second goal of making comments during a play situation, Ethan was observed playing with a special friend from his general education class in the gym. She stood in front of him and said, "Don't forget to talk to me." It was clear that Ms. Hardin had discussed with his peer what Ethan was learning and how the peer could help. The gym was very loud and Ethan was not observed to make any comments. The consultant talked about expanding the activities, perhaps to board games that Ethan knows and likes, in a quiet room with less distraction, especially given that noises were an environmental challenge for him. The team also discussed that his peers may need more ideas of what to say to him so that he could model their comments. One of the issues discussed was having access to typical peers because there was great concern that they not be taken from academics, especially given all the missed days that had interfered with instructional time. The consultant suggested that with more practice and opportunity and use of written scripts, Ethan would learn the skill more quickly. He received a GAS score of −1.5.

Personal Management/Adaptive Skills

Ethan's teacher reported that the third objective of following a relaxation routine and self-calming is going very well. It had become clear to his teacher that changes in Ethan's schedule or things that caused him confusion triggered anxiety. The consultant reminded his teacher of the importance of cueing Ethan early before he became visibly upset and to have him repeat the routine until he was calm. The cue "Ethan, count and blow" has been very effective according to his teacher and parent. The cue card worked well but had to be available and was not always with him. When Ethan was asked if he was calm and he almost always said, "Yes," then he was directed to complete the task on his schedule. His teacher revealed that she had not believed that Ethan could learn to use a relaxation routine to calm down, and she had been pleasantly surprised by his response. Initially, Ethan practiced the routine several times a day, even when he did not need it, so that the cues and the routine became automatic. The consultant reiterated to his teacher that when the skill became rote and automatic, Ethan would be able to perform it on cue when he was beginning to become anxious and upset. He received a GAS score of −0.5.

The time and date for the next coaching was set and the summary report was sent within a week to both the school and parents.

Coaching Session 3

The third coaching session was held a month after the second one, and there had been more snow days for the school. Ethan's mother and teacher were at this meeting; the team viewed a clip of Ethan performing each objective, discussed each objective in detail, and updated the teaching plan if necessary. Ms. Hardin had data for each objective as well.

Communication Skills

The consultant, teacher, and parent observed a video of Ethan answering "wh" questions asked from a peer. At the time of the third consultation, the communication objective of giving full sentences when asked a question about that day's past events was being instructed at least twice a day. Ms. Hardin suggested that they expand the teaching plan to include giving exchanges about home activities. His mother reported that Ethan consistently gave full-sentence responses, and she asked the consultant how to encourage him to give more eye contact during interactions. The group discussed how eye contact was a way to improve the quality of his interactions. Ms. Hardin said she would continue to use peers as well as adults for Ethan to practice full-sentence responses. She would encourage Ethan to ask questions by having possible questions written out for both Ethan and the peer. She would also encourage him to make more eye contact. Ms. Hardin reported that Ethan had spontaneously offered information when he came into school about dinner at Red Lobster. He was no longer using the visual scripts to provide full-sentence information. He received a GAS score of 1.

Social Skills

On the social/communication skill of making appropriate comments during an activity with a peer, the group observed on tape Ethan playing a memory game with a classmate. Both were playing and concentrating but making few comments. Ms. Hardin reported that this skill is worked on twice a day and she is keeping data on the skill. The only change in the teaching plan was to seek out more activities that might be motivating to Ethan and the peers. The team also talked about using video clips to show Ethan and his peers how well they performed. Because Ethan liked to see himself on video, using clips could be a feedback and teaching tool for other skills as well. The consultant discussed the importance of Ethan seeing good examples of himself and others doing the skills. He received a GAS score of −1.5.

Personal Management/Adaptive Skills

On the objective of following the relaxation routine, the team saw Ethan being cued once after he was excited about a toy and did not want to finish his work. He followed the relaxation routine when cued and was able to finish his work. His parent reported that Ethan was able to use the routine at home when cued. This skill was worked on about three times a week when he was getting anxious. The consultant recommended that the teacher and parent update the teaching plan—with Ethan's input—to include a visual list of things that scared or upset Ethan so that he was more aware of when to use the relaxation routine. The consultant also discussed using a visual social story that showed Ethan that when he encountered those things, such as schedule changes or his sister crying, he should use his calming routine of "count and blow." The group discussed cueing him with "What do you need to do?" to help him make the decision himself rather than rely on the direct cue. He received a GAS score of 1.

The final coaching session was set and the summary report was sent to Ethan's parents and teacher.

Coaching Session 4

The fourth coaching session was held about 6 weeks following the third session. There was a 1-week vacation during that time. The consultant met with Ethan's teacher, but his parents were not able to attend because the meeting date had to be changed at the teacher's request. The same protocol was followed. The teacher showed video clips of each of the objectives that were reviewed with the GAS Form.

Communication Skills

The communication skill of using full sentences was worked on about four times a day and Ms. Harden was keeping data. The teaching assistants and peers as well as his teacher worked with Ethan on this skill, and his parents worked on this at home.

Ms. Hardin said that Ethan was responding very well, but that she would like Ethan to begin to initiate questions and comments as well. The consultant and the teacher talked about ways to help him initiate conversation by having topics of interest to him and peers who were responsive. He received a GAS score of 2.

Social Skills

On the second skill of making comments during activities, Ethan was observed in the video clip conversing with another student. Ethan required several verbal cues by adults to remember to comment. It appeared to the consultant that Ethan needed more visual cues such as a list of comments and more modeling from adults and peers. He seemed to not be aware of what to do and was often too engrossed with the activity to remember to comment. The consultant and the teacher also talked about a reinforcement system for both Ethan and the peer such as getting stars that could be exchanged for something of value. The teacher reported that the videotape modeling had not yet been tried. This skill was worked on about twice a day. Ethan received a GAS score of −1.

Personal Management/Adaptive Skills

By the fourth consultation, Ethan needed only one verbal cue for the personal management skill of using a relaxation routine. He was beginning to self-cue spontaneously, saying "Ethan's okay" and not having to go through the routine. He was using this technique about once a week as needed. The teaching plans were updated to include the personal and environmental challenges and personal and environmental supports. He received a GAS score of +2.

Final Evaluation

The final evaluation was done about 6 weeks later. The GAS scores at this time were obtained from direct observation and discussion of data kept. Videotape was made of the observations to allow for the objectives to be reviewed by others. Scores were as follows: Communication +2; Social/Communication +1, Personal Management +2 (Fig. 9.2).

Consultant Comments

The consultant made some observations concerning issues that came up during the consultation. One issue was skill maintenance. The consultant had to continually keep in mind that when a student is making great progress as Ethan did on two of

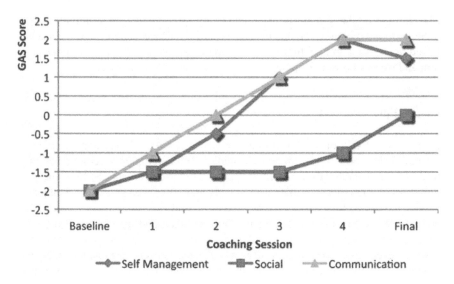

Fig. 9.2 Ethan's GAS scores by coaching session

the skills, a plan is made to ensure maintenance of the skill as well as generalization of the skill and independent performance of the skill so that supports are not eliminated and the skill not maintained. When assessing the skill, the consultant needs to ensure that the teacher provides the supports that are required for success. The amount of time that the skill is practiced and the number of people it is practiced with can make a significant difference in skill attainment. Ethan practiced the two skills more and more often and daily across people over the course of the school year. Some of the problems with the social/communication objective was finding sociable peers with whom to practice regularly and having Ethan and the peer understand what the goal was. More peer training and feedback may have helped and more modeling for Ethan via video clip, social stories, and/or watching peers may have been useful. It also may have helped for the consultant to have modeled peer training and interaction directly. Nevertheless, Ethan exceeded all three of his objectives by the end of the school year.

Case Study 3: Gary

Gary's case study is a shortened description. It begins at Step B. 3. of the COMPASS Consultation Action Plan. Also included are suggested actions to take before reading the teaching plans. Following each suggested action are some possible responses. The reader should review Chap. 3 and be familiar with evidence-based practices and the information provided by the recommended websites.

Background Information

Gary was a 7-year-old Caucasian boy who was diagnosed with autism at the age of 3 years. He attended an elementary school in a rural area of a southern state. At the time of the COMPASS coaching, Gary was a second grader who spent most of his day in general education and the rest of his day in a resource room for additional support. Gary received early intervention services and had special education services since kindergarten. He received speech and language and occupational therapy services at school. Gary was being treated with Zoloft for anxiety.

Gary's parents were divorced. He lived with his mother and two sisters, an 11-year old and a 5-year old. He saw his father on a regular basis. His father worked as an assembly worker and his mother was a childcare worker.

Information from Direct Evaluation

A standardized assessment of Gary's cognitive, language, adaptive, and behavior skills was conducted. Gary received a standard score of 87 for cognitive and problem-solving skills based on the Differential Abilities Scale (DAS). This score fell within the low average range. Gary also had a significant discrepancy between verbal problem-solving and nonverbal problem-solving skills on the DAS. He received a nonverbal general conceptual ability score of 113 and a verbal general conceptual ability score of 54. He received a standard score of 43 on the Oral and Written Language Scales, and a standard score of 65 for adaptive behavior skill composite based on teacher report using the Vineland Adaptive Behavior Scale. Overall, these results indicated that in addition to autism, Gary had significant weakness in verbal problem-solving and communication skills, but also significant strength in nonverbal problem-solving abilities. His adaptive behavior skills were also relatively low and discrepant from his nonverbal intelligence. His teacher completed the Behavioral Assessment Scale for Children, and a T score of 67 was calculated for externalizing behaviors, indicating slightly elevated scores. Lastly, he received a score of 36 from the Childhood Autism Rating Scale, indicating mild/moderate autism.

Step B. 3. Identify and Come to Consensus on Three Prioritized Objectives and Write Measurable Objectives

Three objectives for Gary were agreed upon and written together during the consultation. The objectives were added to his IEP following the consultation. The teaching plans were developed and viewed as continually emerging and changing as his teachers learned more about teaching strategies that worked best with Gary and what environmental supports he needed to succeed. The challenges and supports were taken directly from the discussion of the COMPASS Challenges and Supports

Joint Summary Form completed by his teacher and mother prior to the consultation, as well as from the information obtained from the assessment of Gary's skills completed by the consultant.

Teaching Plan for Objective 1

Objective 1: Gary will engage in conversational turn-taking through four turns (back and forth as one turn) with a peer or small group of peers and in a structured group, staying on topic with visual prompts 4–5 opportunities in a 1-week period.

Personal and Environmental Challenges and Supports for Teaching Plan 1

Personal challenges	*Environmental challenges*
• Has low communication skills	• Has many environmental distractions (verbal, actions, visual)
• Is unable to answer most "wh" questions	
• Has a large gap between his communication abilities and his nonverbal cognitive abilities, which causes him some frustration at times	• Lacks persistent, sociable peers who can entice Gary to communicate with them
• Is occasionally in his "own world" and uses his own scripts	
• Is not that interested in what peers are doing at times	
• Lacks social eye contact	
Personal supports	*Environmental supports*
• Likes computers, games, and age-appropriate TV shows	• Has a team working for him
• Has sisters at home who encourage his interactions	• See teaching plan for specific supports and strategies to teach this skill
• Reads	
• Learns scripts easily	
• Likes seeing himself on videotape	
• Is motivated to interact	
• Has preferences in peers	
• Has emerging social skills	

Suggested Action: Before reading through the plan, consider what methods and materials you would use to teach this skill to Gary. Hint: Refer to Chap. 3 and review the websites on evidence-based practices.

Possible Responses

How would you teach Gary what a conversation means? Does he have the concept of going back and forth on a topic, what a topic is, what listening is and how it looks, or what to say during a conversation?

> 1. Consider whether to begin with an adult, and then consider how to provide training and support to peer(s).
> 2. Consider what visuals to use in teaching Gary.
> 3. Consider how often this can be practiced. The more often, the more likely Gary is to learn the skill.
> 4. Consider consulting with the speech and language therapist and online materials for teaching conversation skills to students with autism.

Teaching Plan

1. Review to the Online Resources for Teachers in the forms section of Chap. 7, especially those on social narratives, video modeling, social interventions, and communication interventions.
2. Use a social story to explain conversations and turn-taking on a topic and why it is important (see Resources for Teachers provided in the forms section of Chap. 7 on how to write a social story).
3. Use a visual chart to teach Gary what a conversation is. There might be topics to choose from, then written comments on one side and questions on another. Experiment to find what works best for Gary to understand and participate.
4. Practice with an adult on choosing a topic, commenting about the topic, and asking questions about the topic. In the beginning, use topics of interest and that he chooses.
5. Show Gary a video of two people having a conversation on a topic of interest to him. Tape Gary having a conversation and staying on topic, and review it with Gary.
6. Expand topics and comments by using visuals.
7. Start with a peer who has been trained, is motivated, and will follow instructions. Use the visuals/scripts with Gary and the peer.
8. Gradually include other peers, one at a time, then a small group. Ensure success with each step.
9. Reinforce Gary with appropriate recognition and incentives and reinforce peers.
10. Practice this at least once a day, two if at all possible, during structured and unstructured activities.
11. Share information with the speech language pathologist and expand activities into sessions.
12. Keep data on progress.

Teaching Plan for Objective 2

Objective 2: Gary will engage in six different turn-taking activities initiated by a peer for 10 minutes with peer prompts only, with each activity reaching criteria four times.

Personal and Environmental Challenges and Supports for Teaching Plan 2

Personal challenges	*Environmental challenges*
• Tends to "be in his world" with emerging interest in what other kids are doing	• Has distractions from competing environmental stimuli
• Has problems keeping focused	• Has limited materials, games, and objects that he is motivated to engage in with others and that are structured with clear beginning and ending
• Has low amount of direct imitation of others	
• Has low motivation to imitate what others are doing	
• Has problems understanding activities without structure of a clear beginning and end of turn-taking	• Has limited time and few motivated peers
Personal supports	*Environmental supports*
• Has many interests that are shared by same age peers (e.g., cars)	• Has a team that is collaborating on his behalf
• Has solid abilities that allow him to do academics in the general education classroom.	• See teaching plan for specific supports and strategies to teach this skill
• Reads, does math, is interested in the computer	

Suggested Action: Consider what strategies to use to teach this skill before looking ahead at the teaching plan that was developed. Remember that teaching plans evolve and change as the skill is taught. Getting input from the school team and from parents and keeping everyone up-to-date are important when plans are adjusted.

Teaching Plan

1. Review to the Online Resources for Teachers in the forms section of Chap. 7, in particular those on social interventions, peer-mediated instruction and intervention, and social skills groups.
2. Select peers and explain the role of a social coach to peer(s). Practice with peer(s).
3. Provide visual supports such as cue card saying "Your turn."
4. Introduce one game at a time and start with games that Gary knows, such as Connect Four or Candyland. Computer games and building/construction activities are other possibilities.
5. Teach Gary the rules of other games before expecting Gary to play the games with a peer.
6. Provide daily practice in a structured lesson.
7. Develop a data system for monitoring progress.

Teaching Plan for Objective 3

Objective 3: Gary will begin and complete familiar work tasks with visual cues and no adult beside him in 4 out of 5 opportunities for 2 weeks.

Personal and Environmental Challenges and Supports for Teaching Plan 3

Personal challenges	*Environmental challenges*
• Is used to adult cues and presence in general education class	• Has distractions around him, competing stimuli
• Is reluctant to try something he perceives as lengthy or difficult and assesses this visually and quickly	• Has tasks that are not familiar or appear too difficult
• Does not ask for help but may ask a question	
• Verbalizes to himself	
• Lacks confidence to work independently and seeks reassurance when working	
Personal supports	*Environmental supports*
• Abilities such as reading, math, fine motor	• Has a team that is collaborating on his behalf
• Likes adult praise	• See teaching plan for specific supports and strategies to teach this skill
• Likes to please	
• Is a visual learner	
• Can reinforce himself/self-monitor	

Suggested Action: Consider what strategies might work best to help Gary learn this skill. What supports does he need to become competent for this objective?

Teaching Plan

1. Review the Online Resources for Teachers in the forms section of Chap. 7: social narratives, structured work systems, visual support, and self-management.
2. Introduce a social story about working by yourself.
3. Have independent, structured work time in an area without a lot of distraction.
4. Start with a task that Gary can do easily to assure success. Make sure there is a clear definition of beginning and ending.
5. Reward starting and completing—not how the work is done—at first.
6. Consider adding a cue card for "I need help" after he understands start and finish so that he knows he can get help and not just stop working.
7. Eventually introduce self-monitoring.
8. Add more than one task when he fully understands and decide on a reinforcement plan.
9. Use visuals to show him his progress and his rewards. For rewards, consider a choice board that is visual and that allows Gary to choose the order of his work tasks.
10. Develop a data-tracking system.

Coaching Session 1

The first session took place about 5 weeks after the consultation with the consultant and Gary's teacher, Ms. Smith. His mother was unable to attend coaching sessions because she could not miss work. Gary's coaching sessions were completed online via Adobe Connect Pro software technology with his teacher at her school and the consultant and support technician at another site. Although this example is based on Adobe software for videoconferencing, it would have been possible to use a web camera with video software such as Skype so that the participants could see each other during the consultation. The only disadvantage with a software program such as Skype is that it does not allow simultaneous viewing of videos and forms. A disadvantage of the Adobe software is that many schools may not have access to it. Thus, an alternative is sending videos of the student–teacher instruction of the objectives on DVDs to the consultant prior to the session or via email.

To observe Gary's current level of performance, his teacher, Ms. Smith, made short videotapes of Gary performing his skills a few days before the coaching date and sent an email to the technician who converted the downloaded footage so that the footage could be viewed using the Adobe Connect program during the coaching session. Written material, such as the GAS Form (replicated on the following page), and teaching plans were shared on screen. Alternately, the forms could have been scanned or emailed to the teacher to download and observe during the consultation if another software program was used that did not allow simultaneous viewing.

Goal Attainment Scale Form for Gary

−2 Present level of performance	−1 Progress	0 Expected level of outcome (GOAL)	+1 Somewhat more than expected	+2 Much more than expected
Has low communication skills and difficulty answering most "wh" questions. Lacks understanding of social skills related to taking turns. Has a conversational script that may relate to his own interests. Not interested in what peers are doing?	Gary will engage in conversational turn-taking through 4 (2) turns (back and forth as 1 turn) with peer(s) or adults and in a structured group, staying on topic with visual prompts 4 of 5 opportunities in a 1-week period	Gary will engage in conversational turn-taking through 4 turns (back and forth as 1 turn) with peer(s) and in a structured group, staying on topic with visual prompts 4 of 5 opportunities in a 1-week period	Gary will engage in conversational turn-taking through 4 (6) turns (back and forth as 1 turn) with peer(s) and in a structured group, staying on topic with visual prompts 4 of 5 opportunities in a 1-week period	Gary will engage in conversational turn-taking through 4 (8) turns (back and forth as 1 turn) with peer(s) and in a structured (or unstructured) group, staying on topic with visual prompts 4 of 5 opportunities in a 1-week period

(continued)

(continued)

−2 Present level of performance	−1 Progress	0 Expected level of outcome (GOAL)	+1 Somewhat more than expected	+2 Much more than expected
Lacks interest in what other kids are doing; keeping focused on an activity is a challenge; does not directly imitate others; has low motivation to imitate or do what other kids are doing	Gary will engage in 6 (3) different turn-taking activities initiated by a peer for 10 (5) minutes with peer prompts only—each activity reaching criteria four times—at least twice a week	Gary will engage in 6 different turn-taking activities initiated by a peer for 10 min with peer prompts only— each activity reaching criteria four times—at least twice a week	Gary will engage in 6 (9) different turn-taking activities initiated by a peer and (make one appropriate comment) for 10 min with peer prompts only—each activity reaching criteria four (6) times—at least twice a week	Gary will engage in 6 (12) different turn-taking activities initiated by a peer and (make at least 2 appropriate comments) for 10 min with peer prompts only—each activity reaching criteria four (8) times—at least twice a week
Is used to adult cues; is reluctant to try things perceived as lengthy or difficult; does not ask for help; has low motivation to complete work tasks	Gary will begin and (or) complete 1 familiar work task during morning work with visual cues and no adult beside him 4 (2) of 5 days for 2 weeks	Gary will begin and complete 1 familiar work task during morning work with visual cues and no adult beside him 4 of 5 days for 2 weeks	Gary will begin and complete 1 (2) familiar work task during morning work (general education) with visual cues and no adult beside him 4 of 5 days for 2 weeks	Gary will begin and complete 1 (3) familiar work task during morning work (general education and resource) with visual cues and no adult beside him 4 of 5 days for 2 weeks

Gary's teacher began the conversation with a discussion about the taping. She reported that she liked being able to tape Gary in his natural setting and view his progress. She also indicated that she intended to use the videotapes for various purposes—to be shared with his mother to show how Gary was progressing and how a skill was being taught, to be shared with other staff members to review teaching methods and monitor progress, and to be shown to Gary (when they were good examples of him doing the skill well) for both reinforcement and review.

The GAS Form, which was developed prior to the first coaching session, was discussed and revised as needed so that Ms. Smith's input and understanding were part of the document. The consultant explained to Gary's teacher that the GAS Form is a tool that helps evaluating learning progress. If progress is not being made, the consultant and teacher must work together to identify what supports need to be changed or added, if more intensity is needed, whether the skill needs to be taught more frequently, what personal or environmental challenges might be interfering with goal attainment, and what personal or environmental supports are not being utilized effectively. After each coaching session, a summary was written and sent to Gary's teacher and mother.

A summary of each of the three objectives is provided below. The observation information, teacher discussion, and GAS rating listed for each objective are described.

Communication Skills

The consultant observed a video clip of Gary having a conversational exchange with Ms. Smith. He was making significant progress with an adult and beginning to better understand how to participate in a conversation. Staying on topic was still a bit difficult for Gary. The consultant suggested ideas that included using a color-coding system for questions and comments that relate to a certain topic; practicing scripts that might be used during a game; using a card to introduce a topic, i.e., "What I had for lunch?"; and a strategy to teach understanding of "topic." The consultant recommended that Gary be given 3X5 inch cards, with some relating to the topic and some not. Gary could be instructed to read the ones that were on topic, which would aid him in learning how to stay on topic. For example, when asked "What did you eat for lunch?," one response might be "I like Candyland." Another might be "I had pepperoni pizza for lunch"; another, "I like to play outside"; and yet another, "I drank chocolate milk." This skill was worked on daily with Ms. Smith, but she had not begun to keep data yet. Gary received a GAS rating of −1 because he is making progress on this skill.

Social Skills

The videotaped observation showed Gary playing Candyland with a peer. Ms. Smith was giving some verbal cues to help keep the turn-taking going, but the boys were involved and attending. Gary's teacher reported that she worked with Gary on this skill once or twice weekly, but had not begun recording data. The GAS form was scored −1 as some progress was being made. The consultant and the teacher talked about other possible activities that could be used taking turns, and Ms. Smith thought that computer access during reading time could be another activity that would work well.

Learning Skills

Starting and completing familiar tasks were observed, and Gary had made significant progress with visual cues. Ms. Smith said she wanted to expand this to other times of the day rather than during Gary's morning work and that she wanted Gary to learn to ask for help as well. The consultant and the teacher talked about creating a cue card that might have written words and a picture illustrating "Raise my hand for help" or "If I need help, I raise my hand and wait quietly for the teacher." A GAS rating of 0, or expected level of outcome, was achieved.

Coaching Session 2

This coaching session was completed about 6 weeks from the last session. There was a 2-week holiday and some snow days between the first and second sessions. Like the first session, this meeting occurred over the internet. His teacher was in attendance.

Communication Skills

By the second coaching session, Gary was starting to demonstrate ability to stay on topic. He used a color-coded visual cue sheet with comments he could make on the topic on one side and the questions he could ask on the other side. He responded well to the materials. He demonstrated staying on the topic and smiled throughout the activity. He had more difficulty asking a question than making a comment, which he was able to do spontaneously. He had some difficulty with eye contact when he asked a question and was instead looking back to the written question to make sure he was saying it correctly. His teacher encouraged eye contact as he learned this skill. Ms. Smith reported that in the morning of the second coaching session, the speech therapist talked with Gary about the community outing he was going on that day. Gary stayed on topic through at least four exchanges with her, and she pointed out to him how well he had done. His therapist was working on this skill also. Ms. Smith has also added a comic strip showing a conversation on a topic to Gary. She felt that he now understood the concept of having a conversation and that a peer who could converse could be added and adult cues faded. He was with peers during speech language therapy. The consultant and the teacher also talked about showing Gary the videotapes of him participating in conversations so he could know how well he was doing and what it looked like. Videotape reviewing would provide both reinforcement and rehearsal for Gary. Examples of other visual supports were also shared. This skill was being worked on more than once a day, as the speech therapist had become involved. Although Gary was making progress, on the GAS Form Gary scored −1.5, as he required many verbal cues from his teacher. However, he demonstrated an understanding of the concept of conversation. The consultant discussed ways to keep data that would be meaningful and not too cumbersome.

Social Skills

Gary was observed during a turn-taking activity with a peer on the computer. Ms. Smith had to give lots of direction and prompting in the beginning because Gary was entering the wrong answer on purpose so he could hear the computer buzz when it indicated an error response. The boys were sitting side by side and sliding the computer back and forth. The consultant and Ms. Smith talked about how to make the interaction more conducive to taking turns. They discussed that the boys should sit across from each other, rather than side-by-side, and encouraged to give eye contact as they acknowledged the change of turns. The teacher reported that Gary also played Candyland and memory games to work on this skill with his general education teacher, resource room teacher, and teaching assistants. Overall, he was making good progress. On the GAS Form, Gary skills were rated at the 0 level or expected level of outcome. Data were now being kept on this skill by his teacher.

Learning Skills

The observation showed Gary reading a book independently. He became engaged in sounding out words and exaggerating the sounds from the words as they would sound if read from a computer. He likes to hear sounds from a computer program even when he knows the word because this is a personal interest. He completed the task and seemed pleased with himself. During the observation, adults walked right by him, and he ignored them and completed his work. This skill is worked on three times a day with his teacher, teaching assistants, and speech therapist. He is working without constant adult cues and doing well. Data are being kept on this skill. The consultant and Ms. Smith talked about introducing the "Help" card in the second grade class because he does not ask for help there and may just sit and wait to be approached. On the GAS form, Gary achieved a +1, as he is now performing the skill in various places and at various times of the day.

Coaching Session 3

This coaching session was completed about 4 weeks after the last session. There were several snow days that interrupted schedules and routines.

Communication Skills

In a video clip, Gary was observed discussing a field trip of going bowling and eating out. Gary answered several questions and remained on topic. At one point, he got a bit silly and said he rode in a roller coaster, but when Ms. Smith asked the question again he answered appropriately. Ms. Smith was pleased with the progress. She had not worked on this skill more than once or twice since the last coaching due to weather and schedule changes. She said she would like to expand this skill so that Gary would ask questions back to the conversation partner. The consultant and Ms. Smith talked about developing some scripts, and Ms. Smith thought that a peer and Gary reading from a script might be a way to start with a peer. The teacher agreed to work on this at least once a day when school resumed a normal schedule. Ms. Smith was keeping data on this skill. The GAS Form was rated at −1 level. The teaching plan was updated to demonstrate the strategies that have been and are currently being used.

Social Skills

Gary was playing a memory game with a peer in the observation. There were many pieces on the table, and it was a long game that lasted more than 10 min. Gary was observed to not only let the peer know when it was his turn, but also he stated when he had a match. He also became excited when his peer made a match. Ms. Smith remarked how nice it was to see him involved with the peer so completely and enjoying the game and his peer. This skill was being worked on daily and data were being kept. Ms. Smith, teaching assistants, and peers worked on this skill with Gary. Ms. Smith said she planned to expand the activities and felt that Gary was making tremendous progress on different turn-taking activities with peers. Ms. Smith was not currently using the "my turn/your turn" card, and Gary was prompting his peers without a cue. The consultant suggested that additional comments he might be taught to make could be, "Great job, you did it, I did it, etc." These might need cue cards at first. On the GAS Form, Gary was at the +1 level consistently. This is more than the expected level and clearly shows how much progress he is making.

Learning Skills

During the observation, Gary was working on a math worksheet about regrouping. He often asked for reassurance by getting Ms. Smith's attention by saying out loud the mathematical computation, e.g., "One plus one, plus one" to indicate whether he was providing the correct calculation. When he would complete the activity, he would smile and sometimes say, "Ms. Smith, I did it." On a few occasions he raised his hand even though he knew the answer. Ms. Smith indicated that this was a less familiar activity, and that when he did it the next day, he completed the activity without any attempts to seek reassurance from the teacher. This skill was worked on a couple of times a day and data were being kept. While observing the video, Ms. Smith said that Gary did indeed need the "I need help" card and that would help him when he was unsure. He raised his hand, even when he knew the answer. The consultant and the teacher talked about the idea of using a card that said, "I raise my hand when I need help and wait quietly for my teacher." After discussion and talking about the data, Ms. Smith said she felt he was at the +1 level overall. The observation, however, revealed that Gary needed more cues on a less familiar task, and the consultant rated him at a −1.

The consultant reminded his teacher that Gary was doing remarkably well, considering the number of snow days and that very little time has passed since the last coaching session. The consultant encouraged Ms. Smith to keep with the teaching plans and the intensity and generalization of the skills. When Gary had more opportunity for learning and he practiced across people and settings, he learned skills well.

Coaching Session 4

This session was held about 6 weeks after the third coaching. Between coaching sessions, there had been a 1-week holiday break and one additional snow day. Compared to the last session, there was much more consistency and time for instruction. The teacher and consultant attended the session.

Communication

In the provided video clip, Gary was observed conversing with a peer. He had a script that he used to ask questions, and the peer had a script to answer questions and ask new questions. The script questions were based on spring break activities and were appropriate and relevant to the students. Gary often did not look at the peer when asking a question, but was prompted by Ms. Smith one time and immediately looked up. He was quite able to converse with adults because adults bore the burden of maintaining the conversation. His strength was responding, but initiating questions using scripting was helping him be more independent. This skill was worked on about four times a day and data were being kept. Ms. Smith provided samples of recent data sheets to the consultant. Ms. Smith, the teaching assistants, and the peers were working on this skill with Gary. The teaching plan was updated. Ms. Smith indicated that she would continue to introduce scripts and would work with this with his peers in regular second grade. On the GAS Form, Gary was rated a 0 and had achieved the expected level on this skill. He also received a 0 for the past couple of weeks from his teacher, meaning that he met this IEP goal.

Social Skills

For the objective of engaging in six different turn-taking activities initiated by a peer, the consultant observed Gary playing with a peer during a game that required each one to take a turn and spell words. Gary needed much verbal assistance to complete the activity. This was an unfamiliar task and the turn-taking activity appeared to be too open-ended. It required him to take a turn and generate a word, then spell it. It was clear that coming up with a novel word was difficult for Gary.

Although his teacher wanted to expand his ability to engage in more complicated turn-taking activities that were naturalistic and representative of what his peers in second grade would be doing, she realized that Gary needed a more structured and familiar activity to continue with this objective as it was written and for him to be successful and feel competent. During the observation, he required verbal cues and help from Ms. Smith. With familiar tasks, however, he is able to play well with a peer. He needed structure and familiarity to be a turn-taker at this point. This skill was worked on three to four times a day and data were being kept on this skill. Ms. Smith said Gary was consistently at the 0 level on the GAS Form. The consultant did not rate the observation because he was not engaged in a structured, familiar activity. Ms. Smith said that she would tape him during a familiar turn-taking activity and send it to consultant for rating.

Learning Skills

During the recorded observation, Gary was cutting shamrocks out of paper in the resource room. He did this activity completely independently and was very proud of his work. When he had finished, he picked them up and showed his work to his teacher. He repeated the praise his teacher said to him several times. A social story has been introduced, but the help card had not been used consistently. Parts of the teaching plan that were important were practicing work time in areas without much distraction, starting with work tasks he could easily do to ensure success and rewarding his starting and completing of work tasks. This skill was worked on about three times a day and data were being kept. It was worked on by everyone in all settings. On the GAS Form, Gary was observed to be at the +1 level by the consultant, and Ms. Smith reported that the +1 level is where he is consistently functioning. Gary exceeded expectations for this goal.

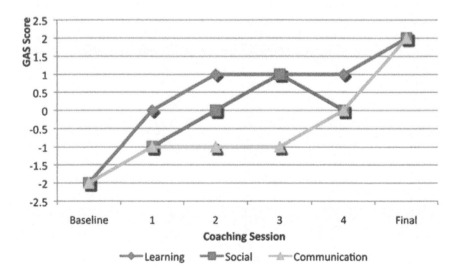

Summary

Ms. Smith was a creative, dedicated teacher who was responsive to the coaching, well prepared, and fully committed to increasing Gary's competency. She kept good data, analyzed the tapes, shared with her staff, and was consistent and positive. Gary responded to all the good teaching. The consultant suggested that at his next IEP, skills could be expanded based on the information collected by his teacher. It also became evident that progress was associated with increasing the number of times and the number of people working on the skill with Gary. The increased time focused on the skills helped Gary learn and retain the skills. However, it is equally clear that Gary needed time to become familiar with a new game, task, or activity before he could be expected to be independent. Gary continued to be followed after the last coaching session (number 4) and at that point was once again videotaped doing the activities and his progress was rated using GAS, which is shown as the final observation on figure of his progress on the objectives over the school year.

Conclusion

In conclusion, the three case studies illustrate both the shared areas of learning common to all students with autism and the unique features that each student and their teacher brings to the learning situation. Although the personal and environmental strengths and challenges for each student were unique, each plan incorporated the use of evidence-based practices for students with autism, ongoing progress monitoring and data collection, and creative problem-solving from the team. A challenge observed throughout the consultations was immediate implementation of all teaching plans and reliable use of data collection. As more research is done in schools, with teachers and students in real classrooms, more answers will be available on effective ways to support teachers and improve educational outcomes for students with autism. Our work demonstrated that COMPASS consultation is effective for improving educational outcomes of students with autism spectrum disorder.

Glossary

Adherence Also called fidelity, refers to how well intervention plans are implemented as planned

Antecedent-based interventions (ABI) Described by the NPDCASD as an evidence-based practice used to reduce interfering behaviors and increase on-task behaviors. Is often used in combination with a functional behavior assessment (FBA)

Adaptive behavior Age-appropriate behaviors necessary for people to live independently and to function safely and appropriately in daily life, such as real life skills of grooming, dressing, being safe, preparing meals, demonstrating understanding of school, community, and work rules, being employed, managing money, cleaning, making friends, socializing, and taking personal responsibility expected of one's age and social group

Behavioral consultation A problem-solving approach that typically involves a consultant and a teacher whose focus is on behavior and whose aim is to design one-on-one interventions to replace a student's targeted problematic behaviors with socially acceptable appropriate behaviors

Boardmaker A software drawing program that is combined with a graphics database featuring more than 4,500 Picture Communication Symbols (PCS) and is commonly used by psychologists, speech pathologists, educators, parents, and others for creating printed symbol-based communication and educational materials

Coaching An ongoing joint activity between a teacher and a consultant designed to assist teachers in the hands-on application of education plans and includes self-evaluation and self-reflection of teaching practices, performance feedback, student progress monitoring, and observation of examples and models of instruction

Collaborative consultation A joint problem-solving activity between a consultant and a consultee(s) whereby all members provide their areas of expertise and knowledge and the solutions that are generated cannot come from one member alone

L.A. Ruble et al., *Collaborative Model for Promoting Competence and Success for Students with ASD*, DOI 10.1007/978-1-4614-2332-4, © Springer Science+Business Media, LLC 2012

Competency The accumulative result of the balance between personal and environmental challenges or risk factors and supports or protective factors associated with specific skills

Computer-aided instruction Described by the NPDCASD as an evidence-based practice and includes the use of computers to teach academic skills and to promote communication and language development and skills. It includes computer modeling and computer tutors.

Consistency The degree to which a student's goal-directed behavior is aligned and in accordance with the teacher's goal-directed behavior for the child (see engagement)

Consultation A problem-solving activity that is indirect and includes a consultant (expert) and a consultee (e.g., teacher; administrator) coming together to generate solutions for an individual student, or for a classroom-wide or a school-wide issue

Consultee The participant who is expected to benefit from the problem-solving efforts involving the consultant

Content skills Refers to the content knowledge necessary for developing competency in specific domains

Context variables Factors that influence the outcomes of consultation may include teacher, student, family, and school variables that need to be taken into account

Control group A group of research participants who do not receive the intervention being studied, but act as a comparison to those who do receive the intervention

Daily living skills Often referred to as adaptive behavior skills, refers to the areas of development that are integral to our everyday routines such as self-care skills (e.g., eating, dressing, bathing), school or work skills, and community skills (e.g., using transportation, making purchases)

Differential reinforcement Described by the NPDCASD as an evidence-based practice and occurs when reinforcement is provided for desired behaviors and not provided for undesired behaviors

Discrete trial training Described by the NPDCASD as an evidence-based practice and is one-to-one instruction used to teach skills in a planned, controlled, and systematic manner, often using task analysis and teaching in small repeated steps

Engagement Refers to the autism engagement rating scale and the need to consider the quality of the child's involvement during learning routines, such as how consistent the child's goal-directed behaviors are with the teacher, how cooperative the child is during instruction, how independent the child is able to perform the skill, how functional the child's use of objects are, how much progress the child makes in a productive activity, and how attentive the child is during instruction

Environmental challenges Risk factors from the environment that hinder learning (e.g., lack of reinforcement)

Environmental supports Protective factors from the environment that encourage or enhance learning (e.g., visual supports)

Experimental group A group of participants who receive the intervention under investigation

Experimental research The gold standard of research that includes method-ological procedures such as random assignment and allows the determination of causality

External consultant A consultant who is brought in from outside of the existing system to consult with the consultee(s)

Extinction Described by the NPDCASD as an evidence-based practice, it is a strat-egy used to reduce or eliminate unwanted behavior by withdrawing or terminat-ing the reinforcer that is maintaining an inappropriate interfering behavior

Fidelity A synonym for adherence and refers to the degree to which an interven-tion is implemented according to its intended procedures

Functional behavior assessment (FBA) Described by the NPDCASD as an ev-idence-based practice, it is a systematic set of procedures used to identify the underlying function or purpose of a behavior and consists of describing the in-terfering or problem behavior, identifying antecedent or consequent events that control or maintain the behavior, and developing a hypothesis describing the likely reason(s) for the behavior

Functional communication training Described by the NPDCASD as an evi-dence-based practice, it is a teaching method, usually associated with FBA, that is designed to replace inappropriate behavior with more appropriate communica-tive behaviors or skills

Goal attainment scaling A systematic measurement system that allows for assess-ment of personalized, multivariable, scaled descriptions of outcome targets that can be used for both process and outcome evaluation

Generalization Refers to the concept that students are able to perform the skill in different environments, with different people and with different cues. It concerns what happens when the teaching plan is stopped or when the student is in a dif-ferent classroom, home, or the community, working with different teachers, us-ing different materials, or interacting with different peers

Internal consultant A consultant who works with a consultee and both of whom are present within the existing system and possess a unique knowledge of the existing structure

Joint attention An early behavioral developmental skill and marker of autism that represents the ability to share one's experience of observing an object or event, by following gaze or a pointing gesture between an adult and an object or event and is critical for subsequent social, language, and cognitive development.

Maintenance The ability to demonstrate a skill over time

Mediators Accounts for the relation between a predictor (e.g., COMPASS consul-tation) and the criterion (e.g., child goal attainment) and helps determine how or why such effects occur

Mental health model Based on the work of Gerald Caplan and refers to consul-tation as a nonhierarchical and voluntary relationship that includes consultee-centered, client-centered, and program-centered consultation, the focus is on work-related rather than personal problems of the consultee, the client's outcome is due to the consultee, and the consultee will learn skills to address similar prob-lems independently in the future

Modeling Providing an example of the behavior you want the child (or the teacher) to exhibit

Naturalistic intervention Described by the NPDCASD as an evidence-based practice and includes a collection of practices such as environmental arrangement, interaction techniques, and behavioral strategies designed to encourage specific target behaviors based on insights into the learner's interests and to provide responses that build more elaborate learner behaviors that are naturally reinforcing and appropriate to the interaction

Nonhierarchical Classified or arranged so that a group or person has the same authority as everyone else

Nonvoluntary consultation In contrast to mental health consultation that assumes a voluntary relationship between the consultant and consultee, other models such as COMPASS does not assume voluntariness as required because the consultee may not necessarily be a volunteer

Parent-implemented interventions Described by the NPDCASD as an evidence-based practice when parents apply individualized intervention practices with their child in their home and/or community

Peer-mediated instruction and intervention Described by the NPDCASD as an evidence-based practice and is used to teach typically developing peers ways to interact with and help learners with ASD acquire new social skills by increasing social opportunities within natural environments

Perceptual motor Skills such as hand-eye coordination, body-eye coordination, and visual-auditory skills that impact play skills, object manipulation, drawing, blocks, and various other forms of physical activity.

Personal challenges Risk factors associated with the target of the consultation, i.e., the child with autism, that hinder learning (e.g., lack of joint attention)

Personal supports Protective factors associated with the target of the consultation, i.e., the child with autism, that encourage or enhance learning (e.g., interest in reading)

Picture exchange communication system (PECS) Described by the NPDCASD as an evidence-based practice that is designed to teach young children to initiate communication with a social partner by giving a picture of a desired item to a communicative partner in exchange for the item

Pivotal response training Described by the NPDCASD as an evidence-based practice based on the principles of applied behavior analysis (ABA) to teach learners by building upon initiative and interests, and is particularly effective for developing communication, language, play, and social behaviors.

Pivotal skills Relates to the idea of pivotal response training and refers to skills that are central to other areas of development, and when promoted, produce improvement in many non-targeted skills and includes responsivity to multiple cues, motivation, self-management, and self-initiations

Presage variables Refers to consultant characteristics that might influence outcomes

Process variables Refers to the specific intervention/training activities (e.g., consultation) expected to have influence on the outcomes

Process skills Consultant skills necessary for effective communication with consultees and includes establishing trusting, collaborative partnerships

Positive behavior supports A function-based system to reduce problem behaviors and enhance prosocial skills through environmental adaptation rather than by use of punishment or other aversive means and includes goal identification, information gathering, hypothesis development, support plan design, implementation, and monitoring

Product variables Outcomes that come from an intervention, can be measured at the student, parent, or teacher level

Prompting Described by the NPDCASD as an evidence-based practice and includes any help given to learners that assists them in using a specific skill

Protective factors Supports that serve to help prevent or reduce the vulnerability of the development or occurrence of negative outcomes

Quality of life A desired global outcome that takes into account the development of competence and the provision of supports that will allow a person to be participating members of society, their community, and their families and includes physical and mental health, education, work, recreation and leisure, and social belonging

Quasi experimental An experimental design similar to a randomized controlled trial, but lacks the element of random assignment to treatment or control. Rather, the researcher controls the assignment to the treatment condition using some criterion other than random assignment.

Randomized controlled trial Considered the gold standard in intervention research, it ensures the highest quality in comparative research designs through randomly allocating participation to receive one or other of the alternative treatments under study

Reinforcement Described by the NPDCASD as an evidence-based practice, it refers to a consequence that follows a behavior which increases the probability that a behavior will occur in the future, or at least be maintained

Response interruption/redirection Described by the NPDCASD as an evidence-based practice for decreasing interfering behaviors, predominantly those that are repetitive, stereotypical, and/or self-injurious and is often implemented after a functional behavior assessment (FBA)

Response to intervention (RTI) An alternative assessment approach designed to evaluate interventions with formative evaluation and obtain data over time to make educational decisions

Reinforce To reward an action or response so that behavior becomes more likely to occur again

Risk factors Challenges that increase the likelihood of vulnerability of the development or occurrence of negative outcomes

Self-management Described by the NPDCASD as an evidence-based practice, it refers to the ability to independently regulate one's own behaviors by discriminating between appropriate and inappropriate behaviors, accurately monitoring and recording one's own behaviors, and rewarding oneself for behaving appropriately.

Single subject design A research design applied to the study of an individual, it is typically used to study behavioral changes in an individual before and after application of the experimental treatment, where the individual serves as her or his own comparison

Social learning theory Based on the work of Albert Bandura, a learning theory that suggests that development of skills can happen from observational learning, imitation, and modeling of others.

Social narratives Described by the NPDCASD as an evidence-based practice that describes social situations by highlighting relevant cues and offering examples of appropriate responding, often includes the use of pictures and other visual supports

Social skills groups Described by the NPDCASD as an evidence-based practice to teach appropriate social interaction skills using direct instruction, role-playing, practice, and feedback

Social validity The social or applied importance of the effects of intervention programs.

Speech-generating devices/VOCA Described by the NPDCASD as an evidence-based practice that uses portable electronic devices that produce synthetic or digital speech and may be used with graphic symbols, as well as with alphabet keys

Structured work systems Described by the NPDCASD as an evidence-based practice developed by Division TEACCH to increase and maximize independent functioning and reduce the frequent need for teacher correction and reprimand through the use of visual supports

Task analysis Described by the NPDCASD as an evidence-based practice of breaking a skill into smaller, more manageable steps in order to teach the skill

TEACCH (Treatment and Education of Autistic and Communication-related handicapped Children) An evidence-based service, training, and research program for individuals of all ages and skill levels with autism spectrum disorders

Time delay Described by the NPDCASD as an evidence-based practice that focuses on fading the use of prompts by giving a brief delay between the initial instruction and any additional instructions or prompts during instruction and is used with prompting procedures such as least-to-most prompting, simultaneous prompting, and graduated guidance

Transactional framework Considers the influence of the reciprocal transactions between a child and caregiver or teacher on developmental outcomes such as language and social skills

Vestibular System The internal physiological mechanisms detecting and contributing to balance in most mammals and to the sense of spatial orientation, movement, and sense of balance

Video modeling Described by the NPDCASD as an evidence-based practice that uses video recording and display equipment to provide a visual model of the targeted behavior or skill

Visual supports Described by the NPDCASD as an evidence-based practice to increase the understanding of language and environmental expectations and facilitates understanding and comprehension by remaining static or fixed in the individual's environment

References

Armenta, T., & Beckers, G. (2006). The IEP: How to meet its demands and avoid its pitfalls. *Principal Leadership, 6*(9), 22–26.

August, G. A., Anderson, D., & Bloomquist, M. L. (1992). Competence enhancement training for children: An integrated child, parent, and school approach. In S. L. Christenson & J. C. Conoley (Eds.), *Home-school collaboration: Enhancing children's academic and social competence* (pp. 175–192). Silver Spring, MD: National Association of School Psychologists.

Bandura, A. (1977). Self-efficacy: Toward a unifying theory of behavioral change. *Psychological Review, 84*(2), 191–215.

Bandura, A., Jeffery, R. W., & Gshedos, E. (1975). Generalizing change through participant modeling with self-directed mastery. *Behaviour Research and Therapy, 13*(2–3), 141–152.

Beglinger, L. J., & Smith, T. H. (2001). A review of subtyping in autism and proposed dimensional classification model. *Journal of Autism and Developmental Disorders, 31*(4), 411–422. doi:10.1023/a:1010616719877.

Bergan, J. R., & Tombari, M. L. (1976). Consultant skill and efficiency and the implementation and outcomes of consultation. *Journal of School Psychology, 14*(1), 3–14.

Billington, T. (2006). Working with autistic children and young people: Sense, experience, and challenges for services, policies, and practices. *Disability and Society, 21*(1), 1–13.

Brown, D., Pryzwansky, W. B., & Schulte, A. C. (2006). *Psychological consultation and collaboration: Introduction to theory and practice* (6th ed.). Boston, MA: Pearson/Allyn and Bacon.

Burns, E. (2001). Developing and implementing IDEA-IEPs: An Individualized Education Program (IEP) Handbook for meeting individuals with Disabilities Education Act (IDEA) requirements (pp. 263). Springfield, IL: Charles C Thomas Publisher. ISBN-0-398-07123-3.

Caplan, G., Caplan, R. B., & Erchul, W. P. (1994). Caplanian mental health consultation: Historical background and current status. *Consulting Psychology Journal: Practice and Research, 46*(4), 2–12.

Castelloe, P., & Dawson, G. (1993). Subclassification of children with autism and pervasive developmental disorder: A questionnaire based on Wing's subgrouping scheme. *Journal of Autism and Developmental Disorders, 23*(2), 229–241. doi:10.1007/bf01046217.

Chakrabarti, S., & Fombonne, E. (2005). Pervasive developmental disorders in preschool children: Confirmation of high prevalence. *American Journal of Psychiatry, 162*(6), 1133–1141.

Cohen, H., Amerine-Dickens, M., & Smith, T. (2006). Early intensive behavioral treatment: Replication of the UCLA model in a community setting. *Journal of Developmental and Behavioral Pediatrics, 27*(2 Suppl), S145–155.

Dawson, G., & Osterling, J. (1997). *The effectiveness of early intervention.* Baltimore: P.H. Brookes.

Dawson, G., Rogers, S., Munson, J., Smith, M., Winter, J., Greenson, J., et al. (2010). Randomized, controlled trial of an intervention for toddlers with autism: The Early Start Denver Model. *Pediatrics, 125*(1), e17–23.

Eckert, T. L., & Hintze, J. M. (2000). Behavioral conceptions and applications of acceptability: Issues related to service delivery and research methodology. *School Psychology Quarterly, 15,* 123–148.

Freer, P., & Watson, T. S. (1999). A comparison of parent and teacher acceptability ratings of behavioral and conjoint behavioral consultation. *School Psychology Review, 28*(4), 672–684.

Guskey, T. R. (1986). Staff development and the process of teacher change. *Educational Researcher, 15*(2), 5–12.

Hurth, J., Shaw, E., Izeman, S. G., Whaley, K., & Rogers, S. J. (1999). Areas of agreement about effective practices among programs serving young children with autism spectrum disorders. *Infants and Young Children, 12*(2), 17–26.

Individuals with Disabilities Education Act. (2004). Retrieved from http://idea.ed.gov/explore/view/p/%2Croot%2C

Jones, K. M., Wickstrom, K. F., & Friman, P. C. (1997). The effects of observational feedback on treatment integrity in school-based behavioral consultation. *School Psychology Quarterly, 12,* 316–326.

Jonsdottir, S. L., Saemundsen, E., Asmundsdottir, G., Hjartardottir, S., Asgeirsdottir, B. B., Smaradottir, H. H., et al. (2007). Follow-up of children diagnosed with pervasive developmental disorders: Stability and change during the preschool years. *Journal of Autism and Developmental Disorders, 37*(7), 1361–1374.

Joyce, B. R., & Showers, B. (1983). *Power in staff development through research on training.* Alexandria, VA: Association for Supervision and Curriculum Development.

Joyce, B. R., & Showers, B. (2002). *Student achievement through staff development* (3rd ed.). Alexandria, VA: Association for Supervision and Curriculum Development.

Lord, C., & Risi, S. (1998). Frameworks and methods in diagnosing autism spectrum disorders. *Mental Retardation and Developmental Disabilities Research Reviews, 4*(2), 90–96. doi:10.1002/(sici)1098-2779(1998)4:2<90::aid-mrdd5>3.0.co;2-0.

Martens, B. K., Hiralall, A. S., & Bradley, T. A. (1997). A note to teacher: Improving student behavior through goal setting and feedback. *School Psychology Quarterly, 12*(1), 33–41.

National Research Council. (2001). *Educating children with autism.* Washington, DC: National Academy Press.

Noell, G. H., Witt, J. C., Slider, N. J., Connell, J. E., Gatti, S. L., Williams, K. L., et al. (2005). Treatment implementation following behavioral consultation in schools: A comparison of three follow-up strategies. *School Psychology Review, 34*(1), 87–106.

O'Brien, S. K. (1996). The validity and reliability of the wing subgroups questionnaire. *Journal of Autism and Developmental Disorders, 26*(3), 321–335. doi:10.1007/bf02172477.

Odom, S. L., Boyd, B. A., Hall, L. J., & Hume, K. (2010). Evaluation of comprehensive treatment models for individuals with autism spectrum disorders. *Journal of Autism and Developmental Disorders, 40*(4), 425–436.

Panerai, S., Ferrante, L., & Zingale, M. (2002). Benefits of the treatment and education of autistic and communication handicapped children (TEACCH) programme as compared with a non-specific approach. *Journal of Intellectual Disability Research, 46*(Pt 4), 318–327.

Prizant, B. M., & Wetherby, A. M. (2005). Critical issues in enhancing communication abilities for persons with autism spectrum disorders. In F. R. Volkmar, R. Paul, A. Klin, & D. Cohen (Eds.), *Handbook of autism and pervasive developmental disorders, Vol. 2: Assessment, interventions, and policy* (3rd ed., pp. 925–945). Hoboken, NJ: Wiley.

Rodger, S. (1995). Individual education plans revisited: A review of the literature. *International Journal of Disability, Development, and Education, 42,* 221–239.

Ruble, L., & Dalrymple, N. (1996). An alternative view of outcome in autism. *Focus on Autism and Other Developmental Disabilities, 11*(1), 3–14.

Ruble, L. A., & Dalrymple, N. J. (2002). COMPASS: A parent-teacher collaborative model for students with autism. *Focus on Autism and Other Developmental Disabilities, 17*(2), 76–83.

Ruble, L., Dalrymple, N., & McGrew, J. (2010a). The effects of consultation on individualized education program outcomes for young children with autism: The collaborative model for promoting competence and success. *Journal of Early Intervention, 32*(4), 286–301.

Ruble, L., & McGrew, J. (2007). Community services outcomes in autism. *Research in Autism Spectrum Disorders, 1*, 306–372.

Ruble, L. A., McGrew, J., Dalrymple, N., & Jung, L. A. (2010b). Examining the quality of IEPs for young children with autism. *Journal of Autism and Developmental Disorders, 40*(12), 1459–1470.

Ruble, L., McGrew, J., & Toland, M. (2010). *Teacher, caregiver, and child predictors of educational outcomes of children with autism.* Poster session presented at the International Meeting for Autism Research, Philadelphia, PA.

Ruble, L., McGrew, J., Toland, M., Dalrymple, N., & Jung, L. (2012). A randomized controlled trial of web-based and face-to-face teacher coaching in autism. Manuscript submitted for publication.

Ruble, L. A., & Robson, D. (2007). Individual and environmental determinants of engagement in autism. *Journal of Autism and Developmental Disorders, 37*, 1457–1468.

Sameroff, A. J., & Fiese, B. H. (1990). Transactional regulation and early intervention. In S. J. Meisels & J. P. Shonkoff (Eds.), *Handbook of early childhood intervention* (pp. 119–149). New York, NY: Cambridge University Press.

Sheridan, S. M., & Steck, M. C. (1995). Acceptability of conjoint behavioral consultation: A national survey of school psychologists. *School Psychology Review, 24*(4), 633.

Sheridan, S. M., Welch, M., & Orme, S. F. (1996). Is consultation effective? A review of outcome research. *Remedial and Special Education, 17*(6), 341–354.

Smith, S. W., Slattery, W. J., & Knopp, T. Y. (1993). Beyond the mandate: Developing individualized education programs that work for students with autism. *Focus on Autistic Behavior, 8*(3), 1–15.

Sparks, G. M. (1988). Teachers' attitudes toward change and subsequent improvements in classroom teaching. *Journal of Educational Psychology, 80*(1), 111–117.

Stokes, T. F., & Baer, D. M. (1977). An implicit technology of generalization. *Journal of Applied Behavior Analysis, 10*, 349–368.

Strain, P. S., Wolery, M., & Izeman, S. (1998 Winter). Considerations for administrators in the design of service options for young children with autism and their families. *Young Exceptional Children*, 8–16.

Thomas, K., Ellis, A., McLaurin, C., Daniels, J., & Morrissey, J. (2007). Access to care for autism-related services. *Journal of Autism and Developmental Disorders, 37*(10), 1902–1912. doi:10.1007/s10803-006-0323-7.

Wahler, R., & Fox, J. (1981). Setting events in applied behavior analysis: Toward a conceptual and methodological expansion. *Journal of Applied Behavior Analysis, 14*, 327–338.

Zirpoli, T. J., & Melloy, K. J. (1993). Behavior management: Applications for teachers and parents. 17(2), 76–83.

Resources on Content Knowledge

Autism Services Research Group. (2004). Compass information series: University of Kentucky: College of Education. Retrieved online www.ukautism.org.

Autism Spectrum Disorder Foundation. (2007). Effective intervention programs. Retrieved online http://www.autismspectrumdisorderfoundation.org/eip.html.

Bebko, J. M., & Ricciuti, C. (2000). Executive functioning and memory strategy use in children with autism: The influence of task constraints on spontaneous rehearsal. *Autism, 4*, 299–320.

Burns, E. (2001). *Developing and implementing IDEA-IEPs: An individualized education program (IEP) handbook for meeting individuals with disabilities education act (IDEA) requirements.* Springfield, IL: Charles C Thomas.

Eggertson L. (2010). Lancet retracts 12-year-old article linking autism to MMR. *Canadian Medical Association Journal*. 182.

Fombonne, E. (2003). Modern views of autism. *The Canadian Journal of Psychiatry, 48*, 503–505.

Grandin, T. (2006a). The great continuum. In *Thinking in pictures* (pp. 33–57). New York: Vintage Books.

Grandin, T. (2006b). *Thinking in pictures*. New York: Vintage Books.

Hale, C. M., & Tager-Flusberg, H. (2005). Social communication in children with autism: The relationship between theory of mind and discourse development. *Autism, 9*, 157–178.

Heward, W. L. (Ed.) (2009) Exceptional children: An introduction to special education. The purpose and promise of special education (pp. 6–47). Columbus, OH: Pearson.

Heward, W. L. (Ed.) (2009). Early childhood special education. In *Exceptional children: An introduction to special education* (pp. 532–563). Columbus, OH: Pearson.

Heward, W. L. (2009). Self-monitoring helps students do more than just be on task. In *Exceptional children: An introduction to special education* (pp. 428–429). Columbus, OH: Pearson.

Howlin, P. (2003). Practitioner review: Psychological and educational treatments for autism. *The Journal of Child Psychology and Psychiatry, 39*, 307–322.

IAN Community. (2011). Therapies and treatments. Retrieved online http://www.iancommunity. org/cs/therapies_treatments/.

Jung, L. A., Gomez, C., Baird, S. M., & Galyon-Keramidas, C. L. (2008). Designing intervention plans: Bridging the gap between Individualized education programs and implementation. *Teaching Exceptional Children, 41*, 26–33.

Koegel, R. L, & Koegel, L. K. (2006). Combining functional assessment and self-management procedures to rapidly reduce disruptive behaviors. In *Pivotal response treatments for autism* (pp. 245-258). Baltimore, MD: Paul H. Brookes.

López, B., Leekam, S. R., & Arts, G. R. (2008). How central is central coherence? Preliminary evidence on the link between conceptual and perceptual processing in children with autism. *Autism, 12*, 159–171.

Lord, C., & Spence, S. (2006). Autism spectrum disorders: Phenotype and diagnosis. In S. Moldin & L. Rubenstein (Eds.), *Understanding autism: From basic neuroscience to treatment* (pp. 1–23). Boca Raton, FL: CRC.

National Institutes of Health. (2011). Developmental Disabilities. Retrieved February 02, 2011, from http://www.nichd.nih.gov/health/topics/developmental_disabilities.cfm.

National Professional Development Center on Autism Spectrum Disorders. (2008a). Session 7: Foundations of communication and social interventions. In *Foundations of autism spectrum disorders: An online course*. Chapel Hill: FPG Child Development Institute, The University of North Carolina.

National Professional Development Center on Autism Spectrum Disorders. (2008b). Session 6: Instructional strategies and learning environments. In *Foundations of autism spectrum disorders: An online course*. Chapel Hill: FPG Child Development Institute, The University of North Carolina.

National Professional Development Center on Autism Spectrum Disorders. (2008c). Session 8: Promoting positive behavior and reducing interfering behaviors. In *Foundations of autism spectrum disorders: An online course*. Chapel Hill: FPG Child Development Institute, The University of North Carolina.

National Research Council. (2001a). Sensory and motor development. In *Educating children with autism* (pp. 93–102) Washington, DC: National Academy Press.

National Research Council. (2001b). Development of communication. In *Educating children with autism* (pp. 45-65). Washington, DC: National Academy Press.

National Research Council. (2001c). Social development. In *Educating children with autism* (pp. 66–81) Washington, DC: National Academy Press.

National Research Council. (2001d). Cognitive development. In *Educating children with autism* (pp. 82–92) Washington, DC: National Academy Press.

National Research Council. (2001e). Adaptive behaviors. In *Educating children with autism* (pp. 103–114). Washington, DC: National Academy Press.

National Research Council. (2001f). Problem behaviors. In *Educating children with autism* (pp. 115–132). Washington, DC: National Academy Press.

Nickels, C. (1996). A Gift from Alex- The art of belonging: Strategies for academic & social inclusion. In L. K. Koegel, R. L. Koegel, & G. Dunlap (Eds.), *Positive behavioral support: Including people with difficult behavior in the community* (pp. 123–144). Baltimore, MD: Paul H. Brookes.

Nounopoulos, A., Ruble, L., & Mathai, G. (2009). An ecological approach to outpatient behavior management services for children with autism spectrum disorders. *Journal of Psychological Practice, 15*, 178–216.

Pretzel, R. E. & Cox, A. W. (2008). Early identification, screening, and diagnosis of ASD, Parts A and B. In *Foundations of autism spectrum disorders: An online course (Session 3)*. Chapel Hill, NC: National Professional Development Center on Autism Spectrum Disorders, FPG Child Development Institute.

Quill, K. A. (Ed.) (2000a). The complexity of autism. In *Do-watch-listen-say* (pp. 1–20). Essex, MA: Paul H Brookes.

Quill, K. A. (Ed.) (2000b). The child's perspective. In *Do-watch-listen-say*. Essex, MA: Paul H Brookes.

Quill, K. A. (Ed.) (2000c). Strategies to enhance social and communication skills. In *Do-watch-listen-say* (pp. 111–160). Essex, MA: Paul H Brookes.

Roselione, B. (2007). Applied behavior analysis teaching strategies: Dan Marino childnett.tv. Retrieved online http://www.childnett.tv/videos/therapies/applied_behavior_analysis_teaching_strategies.

Ruble, L., & Akshoomoff, N. (2010). Autism spectrum disorders: Intervention options for parents and educators. *Communique, 38*, 29–30.

Ruble, L., & Dalrymple, N. (1996). An alternative view of outcome in autism. *Focus on Autism and other Developmental Disabilities, 11*, 3–14.

Ruble, L. A., & Dalrymple, N. (2002). J. COMPASS: A parent-teacher collaborative model for students with autism. *Focus on Autism and Other Developmental Disabilities, 17*, 76–83.

Ruble, L. A., McGrew, J., Dalrymple, N., & Jung, L. A. (2010b). Examining the quality of IEPs for young children with autism. *Journal of Autism and Developmental Disorders, 40*(12), 1459–1470.

Schwartz, A., Shanley, J., Gerver, M., & O'Cummings, M. Answering the question … What are the common qualities and structures of interdisciplinary teams in today's classrooms? Elementary & Middle Schools Technical Assistance Center Extra. Washington, DC: IDEAS that Work: U.S. Office of Special Education Programs.

Smith, S. W., Slattery, W. J., & Knopp, T. Y. (1993). Beyond the mandate: Developing individualized education programs that work for students with autism. *Focus on Autistic Behavior, 8*, 1–15.

Snell, M. E., & Janney, R. (2000). *Teachers guides to inclusive practices: Collaborative teaming.* Baltimore, MD: Paul H. Brookes.

The National Professional Development Center on Autism Spectrum Disorders. What are evidenced based practices (EBP)? Retrieved online http://autismpdc.fpg.unc.edu/content/evidence-based-practices.

Thompson, T. (Ed.) (2007). Disabilities associated with autism spectrum disorders. *Making sense of autism* (pp. 173–185). Baltimore, MD: Paul H. Brookes.

Walther-Thomas, C., Bryant, M., & Land, S. (1996). Planning for effective co-teaching the key to successful inclusion. *Remedial and Special Education, 17*, 255–264.

Wetherby, A. M. & Prizant, B. (2000). The experience of autism in the lives of families. In Autism spectrum disorders (pp. 369–393). Baltimore, MD: Paul H. Brookes.

Wing, L. (1997). The history of ideas on autism: Legends, myths, & reality. *Autism, 1*, 13–23.

Resources on Process Skills

Bramlett, R., & Murphy, J. (1998). School psychology perspectives on consultation: Key contributions to the field. *Journal of Educational and Psychological Consultation, 9*, 29–55.

Buysee, V., & Wesley, P. (2005). *Consultation in early childhood settings.* Baltimore: Paul H. Brookes.

Cormier, S., Nurius, P. S., & Osborn, C. J. (2009). *Interviewing (and change) strategies for helpers* (6th ed.). Pacific Grove, CA: Brooks/Cole.

Egan, G. (2010). *The skilled helper: A problem-management and opportunity-development approach to helping* (9th ed.). Pacific Grove, CA: Brooks/Cole.

Goode T. D. (2009). *Promoting cultural competence and cultural diversity in early intervention and early childhood settings.* National Center for Cultural Competence, Georgetown University Center for Child and Human Development, University Center for Excellence in Developmental Disabilities Education, Research and Service.

Hanft, B., Rush, D., & Shelden, M. (2004). *Coaching families and colleagues in early childhood.* Baltimore: Paul H. Brookes.

Rush, D., & Shelden, M. (2011). *The early childhood coaching handbook.* Baltimore: Paul H. Brookes.

Sheridan, S., & Kratochwill, T. (2007). *Conjoint behavioral consultation: Promoting family-school connections and interventions* (2nd ed.). New York: Springer.

About the Authors

Lisa Ruble earned her Ph.D. in School Psychology from Indiana University. Currently, she is an Associate Professor in the College of Education at the University of Kentucky and Licensed Psychologist. Dr. Ruble was the principal investigator of the two NIH funded studies evaluating COMPASS. She has published over 50 articles in books or professional journals, made more than 100 presentations at international, national, and regional conferences, and consulted and trained hundreds of teachers in autism across Indiana, Kentucky, Tennessee and beyond. She is a past recipient of the New Investigator Award from the National Institute of Mental Health. In 2002, Dr. Ruble established the STAR Program at the University of Louisville and in 1998 helped establish services at TRIAD at Vanderbilt University. Her research program is based on these past experiences when she developed and provided social skills and behavioral interventions, school consultation and training, and parent training. These experiences influenced her interest in services research and the study of issues involved in the provision of evidence-based practices in community-based settings.

Nancy Dalrymple is an educational consultant in the field of autism. She was on the faculty at the University of Louisville School of Medicine, Department of Pediatrics, Weisskopf Child Evaluation Center then became a consultant to the STAR program there. She works with parents and families of children with autism to provide on-going support and information. Nancy also trains school personnel and others who interact with students with autism and has taught university classes. Previously, Nancy was director of the Indiana Resource Center for Autism (IRCA) and was on the Autism Society of America Panel of Professional Advisors as well as other advisory boards. Nancy continues to work with university faculty on research topics. She is the author of numerous research papers and practical source books about autism, and has presented on various topics regarding autism throughout her more than 30 years of experience in the field.

John McGrew earned his Ph.D. in Clinical Psychology from Indiana University. During his doctoral training one of his three primary areas of specialization was autism, for which he extensively utilized the resources of the IRCA, where Nancy was director. Currently, he is Professor of Psychology and Director of the Clinical Psychology Program at Indiana University-Purdue University Indianapolis. Dr. McGrew has been principal or co-principal investigator of more than 15 grants in the area of mental health services. His specialty is in intervention research and implementation science. Dr. McGrew has published over 60 articles in books or professional journals and made more than 75 presentations at national and regional conferences.

Lisa and Nancy first met in 1978, when Nancy was coordinating a residential program for students with autism at the Developmental Training Center (DTC) at Indiana University–Bloomington and Lisa's sister Leslie was in the program. Later, Lisa worked in the DTC program when she was an undergraduate at Indiana University. The program was funded through federal educational grants and was closely connected to the Indiana Department of Education. At that time, the IRCA staff were learning how best to develop programs for people with autism that would help them function in their home communities. Nancy also was a member of the Indiana Legislative Commission on Autism from 1980 to 1994 when the state made significant progress in developing programs for people with autism, including helping to establish the first autism Medicaid waiver in the country. Nancy and Lisa worked together again when Lisa was a master's student at Indiana University-Purdue University in Rehabilitation Psychology and completed her internship under Nancy's direction and her thesis under John's direction. John is now the Director of Training for this same program at IUPUI and during this time became father to Ian, who has severe autism.

Index